Nutrition 101

A Beginner's Guide to Healthy Eating

Park Windsor

Contents

Chapter 1
The Basics of Nutrition

Understanding the Importance of Nutrition

Understanding the importance of nutrition is crucial for maintaining overall health and well-being. Nutrition refers to the process of obtaining, consuming, and utilizing nutrients from food to support bodily functions and sustain life. Here are several key reasons why nutrition is essential:

1. **Provides Essential Nutrients:** Food supplies the body with essential nutrients, including carbohydrates, proteins, fats, vitamins, minerals, and water. These nutrients are necessary for various physiological functions such as energy production, tissue repair, immune function, and hormone regulation.

2. **Supports Growth and Development:** Adequate nutrition is vital for proper growth and development, especially in children and adolescents. Nutrients like protein, calcium, and vitamins are essential for building strong bones, muscles, and tissues, as well as for cognitive development and overall growth.

3. **Maintains Healthy Weight:** Nutrition plays a significant role in weight management. Consuming a balanced diet with appropriate portion sizes helps regulate calorie intake and can prevent excessive weight gain or promote weight loss when necessary. A diet rich in fiber, lean proteins, and healthy fats can help control hunger and support a healthy metabolism.

4. **Prevents Chronic Diseases:** A nutritious diet can reduce the risk of developing chronic diseases such as heart disease, diabetes, obesity, and certain types of cancer. Foods rich in antioxidants, fiber, and omega-3 fatty acids have been shown to have protective effects against these conditions.

5. **Supports Immune Function:** Proper nutrition is essential for a robust immune system. Nutrients like vitamins A, C, D, E, zinc, and selenium play crucial roles in supporting immune function and helping the body fight off infections and illnesses.

6. **Improves Mental Health:** Nutrition not only affects physical health but also mental well-being. Research suggests that a balanced diet rich in fruits, vegetables, whole grains, and omega-3 fatty acids may help reduce the risk of depression, anxiety, and cognitive decline.

7. **Enhances Energy Levels and Vitality:** Consuming nutrient-dense foods provides the body with the energy it needs to function optimally. Carbohydrates are the body's primary source of energy, while proteins and fats provide sustained energy and support various bodily functions to keep you feeling energized and vital throughout the day.

8. **Promotes Overall Well-Being:** Good nutrition contributes to overall feelings of health, vitality, and well-being. When you nourish your body with the right balance of nutrients, you're more likely to experience higher energy levels, better mood, improved cognitive function, and a greater sense of overall satisfaction with life.

The Six Essential Nutrients

The six essential nutrients are the building blocks of a healthy diet, each playing a unique role in supporting various bodily functions and promoting overall health. Here's an overview of these nutrients:

1. **Carbohydrates:** Carbohydrates are the body's primary source of energy. They are broken down into glucose, which fuels the brain, muscles, and other tissues. Sources of carbohydrates include fruits, vegetables, whole grains, legumes, and dairy products. It's essential to choose complex carbohydrates such as whole grains and vegetables, which provide fiber and nutrients, over simple carbohydrates like refined sugars and processed foods.

2. **Proteins:** Proteins are crucial for building and repairing tissues, producing enzymes and hormones, and supporting immune function. They are made up of amino acids, some of which are considered essential because the body cannot produce them on its own and must obtain them from the diet. Good sources of protein include lean meats, poultry, fish, eggs, dairy products, legumes, nuts, and seeds.

3. **Fats:** Dietary fats are essential for providing energy, insulating and protecting organs, absorbing fat-soluble vitamins (A, D, E, and K), and maintaining healthy cell membranes. Unsaturated fats, found in foods like avocados, nuts, seeds, and olive oil, are considered healthy fats and can help lower cholesterol levels when consumed in moderation. Saturated fats, found in animal products and some tropical oils, should be limited, while trans fats, found in processed and fried foods, should be avoided altogether.

4. **Vitamins:** Vitamins are organic compounds that play essential roles in various bodily functions, including metabolism, immune function, and tissue repair. There are 13 essential vitamins, each with its own specific functions and dietary sources. These include vitamin A (found in liver, sweet potatoes, carrots), vitamin C (found in citrus fruits, strawberries, bell peppers), vitamin D (obtained from sunlight and fortified foods), vitamin E (found in nuts, seeds, vegetable oils), and vitamin K (found in leafy green vegetables, broccoli, and soybean oil), among others.

5. **Minerals:** Minerals are inorganic nutrients that are critical for various physiological processes, including bone health, fluid balance, nerve function, and muscle contraction. Essential minerals include calcium (found in dairy products, leafy green vegetables), iron (found in red meat, poultry, beans), magnesium (found in nuts, seeds, whole grains), potassium (found in bananas, potatoes, spinach), and zinc (found in meat, shellfish, legumes).

6. **Water:** Water is essential for life and plays a vital role in numerous bodily functions, including temperature regulation, digestion, nutrient absorption, and waste removal. It makes up a significant portion of body weight and is involved in nearly every physiological process. Staying adequately hydrated is essential for overall health and well-being, and it's recommended to drink plenty of water throughout the day, aiming for at least 8 glasses (about 2 liters) per day.

Macronutrients vs. Micronutrients

Understanding the difference between macronutrients and micronutrients is fundamental to grasping the basics of nutrition. Here's a breakdown of each category:

Macronutrients:

Macronutrients are the nutrients that the body requires in large amounts to provide energy and support various physiological functions. There are three primary macronutrients:

1. **Carbohydrates:** Carbohydrates are the body's primary source of energy. They are broken down into glucose, which fuels the brain, muscles, and other tissues. Sources of carbohydrates include fruits, vegetables, whole grains, legumes, and dairy products. Carbohydrates provide 4 calories per gram.

2. **Proteins:** Proteins are essential for building and repairing tissues, producing enzymes and hormones, and supporting immune function. They are made up of amino acids, some of which are considered essential because the body cannot produce them on its own and must obtain them from the diet. Good sources of protein include lean meats, poultry, fish, eggs, dairy products, legumes, nuts, and seeds. Proteins also provide 4 calories per gram.

3. **Fats:** Dietary fats are essential for providing energy, insulating and protecting organs, absorbing fat-soluble vitamins (A, D, E, and K), and maintaining healthy cell membranes. Unsaturated fats, found in foods like avocados, nuts, seeds, and olive oil, are considered healthy fats and can help lower cholesterol levels when consumed in moderation. Saturated fats, found in animal products and some tropical oils, should be limited, while trans fats, found in processed and fried foods, should be avoided altogether. Fats provide 9 calories per gram.

Micronutrients:

Micronutrients are nutrients that the body requires in smaller amounts but are essential for various physiological processes. They include vitamins and minerals:

1. **Vitamins:** Vitamins are organic compounds that play essential roles in metabolism, immune function, and other bodily functions. There are two main categories of vitamins: fat-soluble vitamins (vitamins A, D, E, and K), which are stored in the body's fatty tissues and liver, and water-soluble vitamins (vitamins B complex and C), which are not stored in the body and need to be replenished regularly through diet.

2. **Minerals:** Minerals are inorganic nutrients that are critical for bone health, fluid balance, nerve function, and other physiological processes. They include both macrominerals (needed in larger amounts) such as calcium, magnesium, potassium, sodium, and phosphorus, as well as trace minerals (needed in smaller amounts) such as iron, zinc, copper, selenium, and iodine.

While macronutrients provide the body with energy and building blocks, micronutrients play essential roles in various biochemical processes, ensuring proper growth, development, and overall health. A balanced diet that includes a variety of nutrient-rich foods is essential for meeting both macronutrient and micronutrient needs and supporting optimal health and well-being.

The Role of Calories in Nutrition

Understanding the role of calories in nutrition is crucial for maintaining a healthy diet and managing weight. Here's an overview of what calories are and their significance:

What are Calories?

Calories are a unit of measurement used to quantify the amount of energy provided by food and beverages. When we consume food, our bodies break down the macronutrients (carbohydrates, proteins, and fats) it contains and convert them into energy to fuel various bodily functions, such as breathing, circulating blood, and physical activity.

Significance of Calories in Nutrition:

1. **Energy Balance:** The number of calories we consume through food and beverages should ideally match the number of calories we expend through metabolic processes and physical activity. This balance is crucial for maintaining a healthy weight. Consuming more calories than the body needs leads to weight gain, while consuming fewer calories than the body needs leads to weight loss.

2. **Weight Management:** For individuals looking to lose, gain, or maintain their weight, understanding calorie intake is essential. By tracking the number of calories consumed and expended, individuals can make informed decisions about their diet and lifestyle to achieve their weight-related goals.

3. **Nutrient Density:** While calories provide energy, not all foods are equal in terms of their nutrient content. It's essential to choose foods that not only provide calories but also offer essential nutrients like vitamins, minerals, fiber, and antioxidants. Opting for nutrient-dense foods ensures that you're getting the most nutritional value out of your calorie intake.

4. **Portion Control:** Paying attention to portion sizes can help manage calorie intake. Even healthy foods can contribute to weight gain if consumed in large quantities. Portion control involves being mindful of serving sizes and listening to hunger and fullness cues to prevent overeating.

5. **Balanced Diet:** A balanced diet includes a variety of foods from all food groups, providing the body with the necessary nutrients while also managing calorie intake. This approach helps prevent nutrient deficiencies, supports overall health, and promotes sustainable weight management.

6. **Physical Activity:** Physical activity plays a crucial role in calorie expenditure. Regular exercise helps burn calories, improve metabolism, build muscle mass, and support overall health and well-being. Combining a balanced diet with regular physical activity is key to achieving and maintaining a healthy weight.

Building a Foundation for Healthy Eating

Building a foundation for healthy eating involves understanding basic principles of nutrition and implementing them into your daily life. Here are key steps to establish a solid foundation for healthy eating:

1. **Eat a Variety of Nutrient-Rich Foods:** Aim to include a variety of foods from all food groups in your diet. This ensures that you obtain a wide range of essential nutrients, including carbohydrates, proteins, fats, vitamins, and minerals. Choose whole, minimally processed foods whenever possible, such as fruits, vegetables, whole grains, lean proteins, and healthy fats.

2. **Focus on Whole Foods:** Whole foods are foods that are as close to their natural state as possible, with minimal processing and additives. These foods tend to be nutrient-dense and provide essential nutrients without added sugars, unhealthy fats, or artificial ingredients. Examples of whole foods include fruits, vegetables, whole grains, legumes, nuts, seeds, and lean meats.

3. **Prioritize Fruits and Vegetables:** Fruits and vegetables are rich in vitamins, minerals, antioxidants, and fiber, making them essential components of a healthy diet. Aim to fill half of your plate with fruits and vegetables at each meal to ensure you're getting a variety of nutrients and promoting overall health.

4. **Include Lean Proteins:** Protein is crucial for building and repairing tissues, supporting immune function, and maintaining muscle mass. Choose lean sources of protein such as poultry, fish, beans, lentils, tofu, tempeh, and low-fat dairy products. Limit intake of processed meats and high-fat cuts of meat, which may be higher in saturated fat and sodium.

5. **Incorporate Whole Grains:** Whole grains provide essential nutrients such as fiber, B vitamins, and minerals. Choose whole grain options such as brown rice, quinoa, oats, barley, whole wheat bread, and whole grain pasta over refined grains, which have been stripped of their nutritious bran and germ layers.

6. **Include Healthy Fats:** Healthy fats, such as those found in avocados, nuts, seeds, olive oil, and fatty fish like salmon and tuna, are essential for heart health, brain function, and hormone regulation. Incorporate these sources of healthy fats into your diet while limiting intake of saturated and trans fats found in fried foods, processed snacks, and fatty cuts of meat.

7. **Stay Hydrated:** Water is essential for maintaining proper hydration, supporting metabolism, regulating body temperature, and flushing out toxins. Aim to drink plenty of water throughout the day and limit consumption of sugary beverages and alcohol.

8. **Practice Portion Control:** Pay attention to portion sizes and avoid overeating, even when consuming healthy foods. Use visual cues such as using smaller plates and bowls, and listen to your body's hunger and fullness signals to help regulate portion sizes.

9. **Plan and Prepare Meals:** Take time to plan and prepare nutritious meals and snacks in advance to help avoid relying on convenience foods or unhealthy options. Batch cooking, meal prepping, and grocery shopping with a list can help streamline the process and make healthy eating more manageable.

10. **Practice Mindful Eating:** Be mindful of your eating habits by paying attention to what, when, and why you eat. Slow down and savor each bite, chew thoroughly, and listen to your body's hunger and fullness cues. Avoid distractions such as screens or multitasking while eating, and focus on enjoying your food and the experience of eating.

Chapter 2
The Food Pyramid and Balanced Diet

Overview of the Food Pyramid

The food pyramid is a visual representation of a balanced diet, illustrating the types and proportions of foods that should be consumed for optimal health. It's designed to guide individuals in making informed food choices and achieving a balanced intake of nutrients. While various versions of the food pyramid have been developed over the years, the most recent model is the MyPlate graphic, which replaced the traditional pyramid-shaped diagram in the United States in 2011. Here's an overview of the food pyramid:

1. MyPlate:
MyPlate is divided into five food groups, each representing a different category of foods:
- **Fruits:** This group includes a variety of fresh, canned, frozen, or dried fruits. Fruits are rich in vitamins, minerals, fiber, and antioxidants. Aim to fill half of your plate with fruits and vegetables at each meal.
- **Vegetables:** Vegetables are an essential part of a balanced diet, providing a wide range of vitamins, minerals, and dietary fiber. Choose a variety of colorful vegetables, including dark leafy greens, cruciferous vegetables, starchy vegetables, and others.
- **Grains:** Grains are divided into two subgroups: whole grains and refined grains. Whole grains, such as brown rice, quinoa, oats, whole wheat bread, and whole grain pasta, are preferred because they retain their nutrient-rich bran and germ layers. Refined grains, such as white rice and white bread, have been processed to remove these nutritious components.
- **Protein Foods:** Protein foods include a variety of animal and plant-based sources, such as lean meats, poultry, fish, eggs, tofu, tempeh, legumes, nuts, seeds, and soy products. Choose lean sources of protein and vary your protein choices to ensure you get a wide range of nutrients.
- **Dairy:** The dairy group includes milk, yogurt, cheese, and fortified soy milk. These foods are rich in calcium, protein, vitamin D, and other essential nutrients. Choose low-fat or fat-free options to limit saturated fat intake.

2. Other Components:

- **Oils:** Oils are not a food group but are included in the MyPlate graphic as a reminder to consume healthy fats in moderation. Choose oils such as olive oil, canola oil, avocado oil, and nut oils, which are high in unsaturated fats and beneficial for heart health.
- **Limit Added Sugars and Saturated Fats:** MyPlate emphasizes the importance of limiting added sugars and saturated fats in the diet. These include sugary beverages, desserts, fried foods, and processed snacks. Instead, focus on nutrient-dense foods and beverages that provide essential nutrients without excess sugar and unhealthy fats.

3. Physical Activity:
In addition to the food groups, MyPlate includes a section for physical activity, reminding individuals to engage in regular physical activity as part of a healthy lifestyle. Aim for at least 150 minutes of moderate-intensity aerobic activity or 75 minutes of vigorous-intensity activity each week, along with muscle-strengthening activities on two or more days per week.

Portion Control and Serving Sizes

Portion control and understanding serving sizes are essential components of maintaining a balanced diet and achieving optimal nutrition. Here's an overview of portion control and serving sizes:

1. What is Portion Control?
Portion control refers to the practice of managing the amount of food you eat in one sitting or throughout the day. It involves being mindful of portion sizes and avoiding overeating, which can lead to consuming excess calories and potentially contribute to weight gain and other health issues.

2. Importance of Portion Control:
- **Weight Management:** Controlling portion sizes can help prevent overeating and manage calorie intake, which is crucial for achieving and maintaining a healthy weight.
- **Blood Sugar Control:** Eating appropriate portion sizes can help stabilize blood sugar levels, especially for individuals with diabetes or insulin resistance.

- **Digestive Health:** Overeating can strain the digestive system and lead to discomfort, bloating, and indigestion. Controlling portion sizes can promote better digestion and overall gastrointestinal health.
- **Nutrient Balance:** Proper portion control allows you to balance your intake of macronutrients (carbohydrates, proteins, and fats) and ensure you're getting a variety of essential nutrients from different food groups.

3. Understanding Serving Sizes:

Serving sizes are standardized measurements used to describe the amount of food recommended for consumption. They provide a reference point for understanding how much of a particular food constitutes one serving. It's essential to differentiate between serving sizes and portion sizes:

- **Serving Size:** Serving sizes are typically listed on food labels and are standardized based on common measurements (e.g., cups, ounces, grams). They represent the amount of food that is considered a single serving according to nutritional guidelines.
- **Portion Size:** Portion sizes, on the other hand, refer to the actual amount of food you choose to eat at a meal or snack. Portion sizes can vary depending on factors such as hunger, appetite, and personal preferences.

4. Tips for Portion Control:

- **Use Visual Cues:** Familiarize yourself with common serving sizes and use visual cues to estimate appropriate portions. For example, a serving of meat is roughly the size of a deck of cards, a serving of grains is about the size of a tennis ball, and a serving of cheese is similar in size to four dice.
- **Read Food Labels:** Pay attention to serving sizes listed on food labels to understand how much food is considered one serving and how many servings are in a package. Be mindful of portion sizes when consuming packaged foods to avoid overeating.
- **Use Smaller Plates and Bowls:** Opt for smaller plates and bowls to help control portion sizes. Research suggests that using smaller dishware can trick the brain into feeling satisfied with smaller portions.
- **Practice Mindful Eating:** Pay attention to hunger and fullness cues, and eat slowly to give your body time to register feelings of satiety. Avoid distractions such as screens or multitasking while eating, and focus on enjoying the taste and texture of your food.

- **Pre-Portion Snacks:** Instead of eating directly from the package, pre-portion snacks into single-serving containers or bags to avoid mindless overeating.

Building a Balanced Plate

Building a balanced plate is a fundamental aspect of healthy eating, ensuring that you consume a variety of nutrients in appropriate proportions. Here's a guide to constructing a balanced plate:

1. Fill Half Your Plate with Fruits and Vegetables:
   - Aim to fill half of your plate with a colorful variety of fruits and vegetables.
   - Choose a mix of different colors and types to maximize nutrient intake.
   - Fruits and vegetables are rich in vitamins, minerals, fiber, and antioxidants, essential for overall health.

2. Allocate a Quarter of Your Plate to Lean Protein:
   - Reserve a quarter of your plate for lean sources of protein.
   - Choose lean meats such as poultry (e.g., chicken, turkey), fish, seafood, lean cuts of beef or pork, tofu, tempeh, legumes (e.g., beans, lentils), or eggs.
   - Protein is essential for building and repairing tissues, supporting immune function, and keeping you feeling full and satisfied.

3. Reserve a Quarter of Your Plate for Whole Grains or Starchy Vegetables:
   - Use the remaining quarter of your plate for whole grains or starchy vegetables.
   - Choose whole grains such as brown rice, quinoa, barley, whole wheat pasta, or whole grain bread.
   - Alternatively, opt for starchy vegetables like potatoes, sweet potatoes, corn, peas, or winter squash.
   - Whole grains and starchy vegetables provide carbohydrates, which are the body's primary source of energy, along with fiber, vitamins, and minerals.

4. Add a Serving of Healthy Fats:
   - Incorporate a serving of healthy fats into your meal to round out your plate.
   - Choose sources of healthy fats such as avocado, nuts, seeds, olives, or olive oil.
   - Healthy fats are important for heart health, brain function, and hormone regulation.

5. Include a Source of Calcium-Rich Foods:
   - Consider including a source of calcium-rich foods in your meal, such as low-fat or fat-free dairy products (e.g., milk, yogurt, cheese) or fortified plant-based alternatives (e.g., almond milk, soy milk).
   - Calcium is essential for maintaining strong bones and teeth.

6. Hydrate with Water:
   - Drink water with your meal to stay hydrated and support optimal bodily functions.
   - Limit sugary beverages, sodas, and excessive caffeine intake.
   - Water is essential for digestion, nutrient absorption, and overall health.

7. Limit Added Sugars and Processed Foods:
   - Minimize the consumption of foods and beverages high in added sugars, refined grains, unhealthy fats, and processed ingredients.
   - Instead, focus on whole, minimally processed foods that provide essential nutrients and promote overall health.

8. Practice Mindful Eating:
   - Pay attention to portion sizes and listen to your body's hunger and fullness cues.
   - Eat slowly and savor each bite, enjoying the flavors and textures of your meal.
   - Avoid distractions such as television or screens while eating to foster mindful eating habits.

The Importance of Variety in Food Choices

The importance of variety in food choices cannot be overstated when it comes to maintaining a healthy diet. Here's why incorporating a diverse range of foods into your meals is essential:

1. Nutritional Adequacy:
   - Different foods contain different combinations of essential nutrients. By consuming a variety of foods, you're more likely to obtain all the vitamins, minerals, antioxidants, and other nutrients your body needs for optimal health.
   - Each food group contributes its unique set of nutrients. For example, fruits and vegetables provide vitamins, minerals, and fiber, while lean proteins supply essential amino acids necessary for tissue repair and growth.

2. Prevents Nutrient Deficiencies:
   - Eating a limited range of foods increases the risk of nutrient deficiencies. For instance, if you only eat a few types of vegetables, you may miss out on specific vitamins or minerals found in other vegetables.
   - Variety ensures that you're not overly reliant on a single source for any particular nutrient, reducing the risk of deficiencies.

3. Supports Gut Health:
   - A diverse diet promotes a healthy balance of gut bacteria, which is crucial for digestive health, immune function, and overall well-being.
   - Different types of fiber found in various plant foods nourish beneficial gut bacteria, helping to maintain a diverse and thriving gut microbiome.

4. Enhances Palatability and Enjoyment:
   - Eating a variety of foods makes meals more interesting, enjoyable, and satisfying. Experimenting with different flavors, textures, and cuisines can make healthy eating more appealing and sustainable.
   - Variety prevents boredom with your diet and reduces the temptation to indulge in unhealthy foods out of monotony or dissatisfaction.

5. Supports Weight Management:

- Consuming a wide range of foods can help prevent overeating by providing a greater sensory experience and satisfying diverse taste preferences.
- Including a variety of nutrient-dense foods in your diet helps keep you feeling full and satisfied, reducing the likelihood of excessive calorie intake and supporting weight management efforts.

6. Reduces Exposure to Toxins and Contaminants:
- Consuming a diverse range of foods helps mitigate the risk of overexposure to potentially harmful substances, such as pesticides, heavy metals, and environmental toxins.
- Eating a variety of foods from different sources and regions helps diversify your exposure to potential contaminants, minimizing potential health risks.

7. Promotes Culinary Creativity and Skill Development:
- Exploring diverse foods and cuisines encourages culinary creativity and expands your cooking skills.
- Trying new ingredients and recipes can broaden your culinary repertoire, making meal preparation more enjoyable and satisfying.

Adapting the Food Pyramid to Individual Needs

Adapting the food pyramid to individual needs involves customizing dietary recommendations based on factors such as age, gender, activity level, health status, and personal preferences. While the food pyramid provides general guidelines for building a balanced diet, it's essential to tailor these recommendations to meet individual nutritional requirements and goals. Here's how to adapt the food pyramid to individual needs:

1. Consider Caloric Needs:
- Caloric needs vary based on factors such as age, gender, weight, height, and activity level. Individuals with higher energy requirements, such as athletes or those with physically demanding jobs, may need larger portions or more frequent meals to meet their calorie needs.
- Adjust portion sizes and food choices accordingly to ensure adequate energy intake while maintaining a balanced diet.

2. Customize Macronutrient Ratios:

- The recommended distribution of macronutrients (carbohydrates, proteins, and fats) can vary depending on individual goals and preferences.
- For example, athletes or individuals engaging in intense physical activity may benefit from a higher proportion of carbohydrates to support energy levels and performance.
- Those following specific dietary patterns, such as low-carb or high-protein diets, should adjust their macronutrient ratios accordingly while still ensuring a balance of nutrients.

3. Consider Dietary Restrictions and Preferences:

- Individuals with food allergies, intolerances, or specific dietary restrictions (e.g., vegetarian, vegan, gluten-free) need to adapt their food choices accordingly.
- Substitute alternative sources of nutrients to meet dietary restrictions while still ensuring a balanced intake of essential nutrients.
- Take into account personal preferences, cultural influences, and ethical considerations when planning meals and making food choices.

4. Address Specific Health Needs:

- Individuals with certain health conditions, such as diabetes, heart disease, hypertension, or gastrointestinal disorders, may require dietary modifications to manage their condition effectively.
- Consult with a healthcare provider or registered dietitian to develop a personalized nutrition plan tailored to specific health needs and goals.
- Consider factors such as sodium, sugar, and saturated fat intake, as well as nutrient density and portion control, when adapting the food pyramid to address health concerns.

5. Plan for Age-Related Needs:

- Nutritional requirements change throughout the lifecycle, with specific needs during infancy, childhood, adolescence, adulthood, and older age.
- Adapt the food pyramid to meet age-related needs, such as increased calcium and vitamin D intake for bone health in adolescents

and older adults, or higher protein intake for muscle maintenance in older adults.

6. Monitor and Adjust:
- Regularly assess dietary habits, nutritional intake, and health status to ensure that dietary needs are being met.
- Be flexible and willing to adjust dietary recommendations based on changes in lifestyle, health status, or personal preferences.

Chapter 3
The Power of Whole
Foods

Defining Whole Foods

Whole foods refer to foods that are in their natural, unprocessed state or have undergone minimal processing and refining. These foods are typically nutrient-dense and contain a variety of essential vitamins, minerals, fiber, and other beneficial compounds. Here's a more detailed definition of whole foods:

1. Unprocessed or Minimally Processed:

- Whole foods are either in their natural state or have undergone minimal processing to preserve their nutritional integrity. They are not heavily refined or altered from their original form.
- Examples of unprocessed or minimally processed whole foods include fresh fruits and vegetables, whole grains, legumes, nuts, seeds, eggs, poultry, fish, and lean meats.

2. Nutrient-Dense:

- Whole foods are rich in essential nutrients, providing a wide range of vitamins, minerals, antioxidants, phytochemicals, and dietary fiber.
- These nutrients are naturally occurring and are not added during processing or fortification.

3. No Added Sugars, Salt, or Artificial Ingredients:

- Whole foods do not contain added sugars, salt, artificial flavors, colors, or preservatives. They are free from synthetic additives commonly found in processed and packaged foods.
- By avoiding added sugars and excessive salt, whole foods support overall health and reduce the risk of chronic diseases such as obesity, diabetes, and heart disease.

4. Examples of Whole Foods:

- Fruits and Vegetables: Fresh or frozen fruits and vegetables, including berries, leafy greens, cruciferous vegetables, citrus fruits, and root vegetables.
- Whole Grains: Whole grains such as brown rice, quinoa, oats, barley, whole wheat, bulgur, millet, and farro.
- Legumes: Beans, lentils, chickpeas, peas, and soybeans are rich sources of protein, fiber, vitamins, and minerals.

- Nuts and Seeds: Almonds, walnuts, peanuts, chia seeds, flaxseeds, pumpkin seeds, and sunflower seeds provide healthy fats, protein, and essential nutrients.
- Lean Proteins: Poultry, fish, seafood, eggs, tofu, tempeh, and legumes are nutritious sources of protein and other essential nutrients.
- Dairy: Plain yogurt, milk, cheese, and cottage cheese without added sugars or artificial ingredients.
- Herbs and Spices: Fresh or dried herbs and spices add flavor and nutritional value to meals without added calories, sodium, or artificial additives.

5. Benefits of Whole Foods:
- Improved Nutrient Intake: Whole foods provide a wide range of essential nutrients, promoting overall health and well-being.
- Satiety and Weight Management: Whole foods are often more filling and satisfying than processed foods, helping to control appetite and support weight management.
- Reduced Risk of Chronic Diseases: Consuming a diet rich in whole foods is associated with a lower risk of chronic diseases such as heart disease, diabetes, and certain cancers.
- Enhanced Digestive Health: Whole foods are high in dietary fiber, which supports digestive health, regularity, and gut microbiome diversity.

Benefits of Whole Foods over Processed Foods

Whole foods offer numerous advantages over processed foods when it comes to supporting overall health and well-being. Here are some key benefits of choosing whole foods over processed foods:

1. Nutrient Density:
- Whole foods are naturally rich in essential nutrients, including vitamins, minerals, antioxidants, fiber, and phytochemicals. These nutrients are essential for various bodily functions, such as metabolism, immune function, and tissue repair.
- Processed foods, on the other hand, are often stripped of nutrients during processing and may contain added sugars, unhealthy fats, and artificial additives.

2. Higher Fiber Content:

- Whole foods, such as fruits, vegetables, whole grains, legumes, nuts, and seeds, are excellent sources of dietary fiber. Fiber promotes digestive health, helps regulate blood sugar levels, and supports weight management by increasing feelings of fullness and reducing calorie intake.
- Processed foods, especially those made with refined grains and added sugars, tend to be low in fiber and may contribute to digestive issues and blood sugar spikes.

3. Lower in Added Sugars and Sodium:

- Whole foods are free from added sugars, excessive sodium, artificial sweeteners, and preservatives commonly found in processed foods. Excessive intake of added sugars and sodium is linked to various health problems, including obesity, diabetes, heart disease, and hypertension.
- By choosing whole foods, you can better control your intake of sugars and sodium, supporting overall health and reducing the risk of chronic diseases.

4. Reduced Caloric Density:

- Whole foods are generally lower in calories and higher in volume compared to processed foods. This means you can consume larger portions of whole foods while still managing your calorie intake, promoting feelings of satiety and satisfaction.
- Processed foods, particularly those high in added sugars, unhealthy fats, and refined carbohydrates, are often calorie-dense and can contribute to excessive calorie consumption and weight gain.

5. Supports Sustainable Weight Management:

- Incorporating whole foods into your diet can support sustainable weight management by providing essential nutrients, promoting satiety, and reducing cravings for processed foods.
- Whole foods are less likely to contribute to overeating and weight gain compared to processed foods, which may lead to better long-term adherence to a healthy eating plan.

6. Improved Flavor and Culinary Experience:

- Whole foods offer vibrant flavors, textures, and aromas that enhance the culinary experience. Cooking with fresh ingredients allows you to experiment with different recipes, herbs, and spices, creating delicious and nutritious meals.
- Processed foods often contain artificial flavors, additives, and preservatives to enhance taste and shelf life, but they lack the complexity and freshness of whole foods.

7. Supports Environmental Sustainability:
- Choosing whole foods over processed foods can have positive environmental impacts by reducing the demand for highly processed and packaged products.
- Whole foods, especially plant-based options, require fewer resources such as water, land, and energy to produce compared to processed foods, which often involve extensive manufacturing and packaging processes.

Incorporating Whole Grains in Your Diet

Incorporating whole grains into your diet is a simple yet effective way to boost your intake of essential nutrients, fiber, and antioxidants while promoting overall health. Here are some tips for incorporating whole grains into your meals:

1. Choose Whole Grain Varieties:
- When selecting grains, opt for whole grain options such as brown rice, quinoa, oats, barley, whole wheat, bulgur, millet, and farro.
- Check food labels and ingredient lists to ensure that the product contains whole grains as the first ingredient. Look for terms like "whole wheat," "whole grain," "whole oats," or "whole rye."

2. Start Your Day with Whole Grains:
- Enjoy whole grain cereals or oatmeal for breakfast. Look for unsweetened options and add fresh fruit, nuts, seeds, or a drizzle of honey for extra flavor and nutrition.
- Substitute refined grains with whole grain options in breakfast foods such as pancakes, waffles, and muffins.

3. Incorporate Whole Grains into Baked Goods:

- Use whole wheat flour or other whole grain flours in baking recipes for bread, pizza dough, muffins, cookies, and cakes.
- Experiment with different whole grain flours such as whole wheat, spelt, buckwheat, or almond flour to add variety to your baked goods.

4. Bulk Up Salads and Soups:

- Add cooked whole grains like quinoa, bulgur, barley, or brown rice to salads and soups to increase their nutritional content and make them more filling.
- Whole grains add texture, flavor, and fiber to salads and soups, making them satisfying and nutritious meal options.

5. Substitute Whole Grains for Refined Grains:

- Replace refined grains with whole grain alternatives in your favorite recipes. For example, use brown rice instead of white rice, whole wheat pasta instead of regular pasta, or whole grain bread instead of white bread.
- Gradually transition to whole grain options in your meals to adapt to the different taste and texture.

6. Snack on Whole Grain Options:

- Choose whole grain snacks such as air-popped popcorn, whole grain crackers, whole grain rice cakes, or whole grain cereal bars.
- Look for snacks with minimal added sugars and unhealthy fats and opt for whole grain options for sustained energy and satiety.

7. Experiment with Ancient Grains:

- Explore ancient grains such as quinoa, farro, bulgur, amaranth, teff, and spelt to add variety to your meals.
- These grains offer unique flavors, textures, and nutritional profiles and can be used in a variety of dishes, from salads and pilafs to porridges and baked goods.

8. Read Labels and Ingredient Lists:

- Pay attention to food labels and ingredient lists when purchasing packaged foods to ensure they contain whole grains.
- Look for products with whole grains listed as the first ingredient and avoid those with refined grains, added sugars, and unhealthy fats.

Choosing Fresh Fruits and Vegetables

Choosing fresh fruits and vegetables is an excellent way to incorporate nutrient-dense foods into your diet and reap numerous health benefits. Here's how to select and incorporate fresh produce into your meals:

1. Opt for Seasonal Produce:
   - Choose fruits and vegetables that are in season for the freshest and most flavorful options. Seasonal produce tends to be more abundant, affordable, and nutritious.
   - Visit farmers' markets or local produce stands to find a variety of seasonal fruits and vegetables grown in your region.

2. Select a Variety of Colors:
   - Aim to include a rainbow of colors in your fruit and vegetable selection. Different colors indicate the presence of various vitamins, minerals, antioxidants, and phytonutrients.
   - Choose a mix of vibrant fruits and vegetables such as leafy greens, red bell peppers, orange carrots, purple eggplants, yellow squash, and blueberries to maximize nutrient intake.

3. Consider Texture and Ripeness:
   - Look for fruits and vegetables that are firm, vibrant in color, and free from bruises, blemishes, or signs of decay. Avoid produce that feels mushy or has moldy spots.
   - Choose ripe fruits and vegetables that are ready to eat or slightly underripe, as they will continue to ripen at home. Check for ripeness by gently pressing or smelling the produce.

4. Pay Attention to Seasoning and Smell:
   - Use your senses to assess the freshness and quality of fruits and vegetables. Fresh produce should have a pleasant aroma and smell fragrant and ripe.
   - Avoid fruits and vegetables that have an off-putting odor or smell sour, musty, or rotten, as they may be past their prime or spoiled.

5. Consider Organic Options:

- If possible, choose organic fruits and vegetables to minimize exposure to pesticides, synthetic fertilizers, and other harmful chemicals.
   - Refer to the Environmental Working Group's "Dirty Dozen" list to prioritize organic options for produce with higher pesticide residues, such as strawberries, spinach, apples, and bell peppers.

6. Buy Local and Support Sustainable Practices:
   - Support local farmers and sustainable agricultural practices by purchasing locally grown fruits and vegetables.
   - Local produce is often fresher, tastier, and more environmentally friendly than imported options, as it requires fewer resources for transportation and storage.

7. Store Properly to Maintain Freshness:
   - Store fruits and vegetables properly to prolong freshness and prevent spoilage. Some produce items, such as berries and leafy greens, are best stored in the refrigerator, while others, like tomatoes and bananas, are better kept at room temperature.
   - Use crisper drawers, produce bags, or containers to keep fruits and vegetables fresh and organized in the refrigerator.

8. Incorporate Fresh Produce into Every Meal:
   - Include fresh fruits and vegetables in every meal and snack throughout the day. Add sliced bananas or berries to oatmeal, top salads with a variety of colorful vegetables, and enjoy fresh fruit as a snack or dessert.
   - Experiment with different cooking methods, such as roasting, grilling, steaming, or sautéing, to enhance the flavor and texture of fresh produce.

The Role of Lean Proteins in Whole Food Nutrition

Lean proteins play a crucial role in whole food nutrition by providing essential nutrients, supporting muscle growth and repair, and promoting overall health and well-being. Here's a closer look at the role of lean proteins in whole food nutrition:

1. Essential Amino Acids:
 - Proteins are made up of amino acids, some of which are essential, meaning they must be obtained from the diet because the body cannot produce them.
 - Lean proteins, such as poultry, fish, eggs, tofu, legumes, and low-fat dairy products, provide a complete or high-quality source of essential amino acids necessary for various bodily functions, including protein synthesis, tissue repair, and immune function.

2. Muscle Growth and Repair:
 - Protein is essential for building and repairing muscle tissue, making it particularly important for individuals engaged in physical activity, exercise, or strength training.
 - Consuming lean proteins after exercise helps support muscle recovery, repair damaged tissues, and promote muscle growth and strength.

3. Satiety and Weight Management:
 - Protein is the most satiating macronutrient, meaning it helps keep you feeling full and satisfied after meals, reducing hunger and cravings.
 - Incorporating lean proteins into meals and snacks can help control appetite, regulate food intake, and support weight management efforts by reducing overall calorie consumption.

4. Nutrient Density:
 - Lean proteins are nutrient-dense foods, meaning they provide a high concentration of essential nutrients relative to their calorie content.
 - In addition to amino acids, lean proteins are rich in vitamins, minerals, and other bioactive compounds that support overall health and well-being.

5. Heart Health:
 - Choosing lean proteins over higher-fat options can help reduce intake of saturated and trans fats, which are linked to an increased risk of heart disease.
 - Lean proteins such as poultry, fish, and plant-based sources like legumes and tofu are lower in saturated fat and cholesterol compared to fatty cuts of meat and processed meats.

6. Blood Sugar Control:

- Protein-rich foods have a minimal impact on blood sugar levels compared to carbohydrates, helping to stabilize blood glucose levels and prevent spikes and crashes.
- Including lean proteins in meals and snacks can help balance macronutrient intake, improve glycemic control, and reduce the risk of insulin resistance and type 2 diabetes.

7. Variety and Flexibility:

- Lean proteins come in a variety of options, allowing for flexibility and customization in meal planning and food choices.
- Whether you prefer animal-based proteins like chicken, turkey, fish, and eggs, or plant-based options such as tofu, tempeh, legumes, and lentils, there are numerous lean protein sources to suit different dietary preferences and needs.

8. Sustainable and Ethical Choices:

- Choosing lean proteins from sustainable and ethically sourced sources supports environmentally friendly practices and animal welfare.
- Look for labels such as organic, pasture-raised, wild-caught, or grass-fed to ensure you're making environmentally conscious and humane choices when selecting lean protein options.

Chapter 4
Understanding Macronutrients

Carbohydrates: Types and Sources

Carbohydrates are one of the three main macronutrients, along with proteins and fats, and they serve as the primary source of energy for the body. Understanding the different types and sources of carbohydrates is essential for making informed dietary choices. Here's an overview:

1. Simple Carbohydrates:
   - Simple carbohydrates, also known as sugars, are composed of one or two sugar molecules and are quickly digested and absorbed into the bloodstream, leading to rapid spikes in blood sugar levels.
   - Sources of simple carbohydrates include:
   - **Natural Sources:** Fruits (e.g., bananas, grapes, oranges), vegetables (e.g., carrots, beets), and dairy products (e.g., milk, yogurt) contain naturally occurring sugars such as fructose and lactose.
   - **Added Sugars:** Processed and packaged foods often contain added sugars, such as sucrose, glucose, and high-fructose corn syrup, which contribute to sweetness and flavor. Examples include candies, sodas, pastries, and sweetened beverages.
   - **Refined Grains:** Refined grains, such as white flour, white rice, and products made with white flour (e.g., white bread, pasta), have been processed to remove the bran and germ, stripping away fiber and nutrients.

2. Complex Carbohydrates:
   - Complex carbohydrates consist of longer chains of sugar molecules and take longer to digest, resulting in a slower and more sustained release of energy.
   - Sources of complex carbohydrates include:
   - **Whole Grains:** Whole grains contain all parts of the grain, including the bran, germ, and endosperm, providing fiber, vitamins, minerals, and antioxidants. Examples include brown rice, quinoa, oats, barley, whole wheat bread, and whole grain pasta.
   - **Legumes:** Legumes, such as beans (e.g., black beans, kidney beans, chickpeas), lentils, and peas, are rich sources of complex carbohydrates, protein, fiber, and micronutrients.

- **Starchy Vegetables:** Starchy vegetables like potatoes, sweet potatoes, corn, peas, and winter squash are high in complex carbohydrates, vitamins, and minerals.
- **Fiber-Rich Foods:** High-fiber foods, such as bran cereals, whole fruits, vegetables, and nuts, contain complex carbohydrates that provide bulk, promote satiety, and support digestive health.

3. Dietary Fiber:
- Dietary fiber is a type of carbohydrate found in plant foods that cannot be digested by the body but plays a crucial role in digestive health, blood sugar control, and weight management.
- Sources of dietary fiber include whole grains, fruits, vegetables, legumes, nuts, and seeds.
- Soluble fiber, found in foods like oats, beans, and fruits, dissolves in water and forms a gel-like substance in the digestive tract, helping to lower cholesterol levels and stabilize blood sugar.
- Insoluble fiber, found in foods like wheat bran, vegetables, and nuts, adds bulk to stools and promotes regularity by aiding in the movement of food through the digestive system.

4. Glycemic Index:
- The glycemic index (GI) is a measure of how quickly and significantly a carbohydrate-containing food raises blood sugar levels.
- Foods with a high GI cause a rapid spike in blood sugar, while those with a low GI lead to a slower and more gradual increase in blood sugar.
- Choosing foods with a lower glycemic index, such as whole grains, legumes, and non-starchy vegetables, can help stabilize blood sugar levels, reduce hunger, and promote overall health.

Proteins: Essential Building Blocks

Proteins are essential macronutrients that serve as the building blocks for tissues, muscles, enzymes, hormones, and other vital components of the body. Understanding the importance of proteins and their role in the diet is crucial for maintaining overall health and well-being. Here's an overview of proteins as essential building blocks:

1. Structural Component of Cells and Tissues:

- Proteins are the main structural component of cells, tissues, and organs in the body. They form the framework that gives structure, strength, and support to muscles, bones, skin, hair, nails, and internal organs.
- Collagen, a type of structural protein, is abundant in connective tissues such as tendons, ligaments, cartilage, and skin, providing strength and elasticity.

2. Muscle Growth and Repair:

- Proteins play a crucial role in muscle growth, repair, and maintenance. During exercise, physical activity, or periods of growth, proteins are broken down into amino acids, which are used to repair damaged muscle tissues and build new muscle fibers.
- Consuming adequate protein from dietary sources is essential for supporting muscle recovery, strength, and performance, especially for individuals engaged in resistance training or endurance exercise.

3. Enzymes and Hormones:

- Proteins serve as enzymes, which are biological catalysts that facilitate chemical reactions in the body. Enzymes are involved in various metabolic processes, including digestion, energy production, and detoxification.
- Hormones, such as insulin, glucagon, and growth hormone, are protein-based molecules that regulate physiological functions, metabolism, growth, and development.

4. Immune Function and Defense:

- Proteins are essential for maintaining a healthy immune system and defending the body against pathogens, viruses, and foreign invaders.
- Antibodies, which are specialized proteins produced by the immune system, recognize and neutralize harmful substances, pathogens, and toxins, helping to prevent infections and illness.

5. Transport and Storage:

- Proteins serve as carriers and transport molecules, facilitating the movement of nutrients, oxygen, hormones, and other substances throughout the body.

- Hemoglobin, a protein found in red blood cells, transports oxygen from the lungs to tissues and organs, while myoglobin stores oxygen in muscle cells for energy production during exercise.

6. pH Balance and Acid-Base Regulation:
  - Proteins help maintain acid-base balance and pH levels in the body by acting as buffers and stabilizing internal pH.
  - Proteins can accept or donate hydrogen ions (H+) to regulate pH and prevent shifts in acidity or alkalinity, which are critical for optimal cellular function and metabolic processes.

7. Source of Essential Amino Acids:
  - Proteins are composed of amino acids, some of which are essential, meaning they cannot be synthesized by the body and must be obtained from the diet.
  - Dietary proteins provide essential amino acids necessary for protein synthesis, tissue repair, and various physiological functions.

8. Dietary Sources of Protein:
  - Protein-rich foods include animal-based sources such as lean meats, poultry, fish, eggs, dairy products (e.g., milk, yogurt, cheese), and plant-based sources such as legumes (e.g., beans, lentils, chickpeas), tofu, tempeh, seitan, nuts, seeds, and whole grains.

Fats: Types and Healthy Choices

Fats are essential macronutrients that play various roles in the body, including providing energy, supporting cell structure, and aiding in the absorption of fat-soluble vitamins. Understanding the different types of fats and making healthy choices is crucial for maintaining overall health and well-being. Here's an overview of fats, their types, and healthy choices:

1. Types of Fats:
  - **Saturated Fats:** Saturated fats are typically solid at room temperature and are found in animal products such as meat, dairy, and butter, as well as certain plant oils like coconut oil and palm oil. While saturated fats can raise LDL (bad) cholesterol levels when consumed in

excess, they also play essential roles in hormone production and cell membrane structure.

- **Monounsaturated Fats:** Monounsaturated fats are liquid at room temperature and are found in foods such as olive oil, avocados, nuts, and seeds. Consuming monounsaturated fats in place of saturated fats may help improve cholesterol levels and reduce the risk of heart disease.

- **Polyunsaturated Fats:** Polyunsaturated fats are also liquid at room temperature and include omega-3 and omega-6 fatty acids. Sources of omega-3 fatty acids include fatty fish (e.g., salmon, mackerel, sardines), flaxseeds, chia seeds, walnuts, and algae. Omega-6 fatty acids are found in vegetable oils (e.g., soybean oil, corn oil, sunflower oil), nuts, and seeds. Both omega-3 and omega-6 fatty acids are essential for brain function, heart health, and inflammation regulation.

- **Trans Fats:** Trans fats are artificially produced through hydrogenation, a process that converts liquid vegetable oils into solid fats. Trans fats are found in partially hydrogenated oils used in processed and fried foods, baked goods, and margarine. Consuming trans fats can raise LDL cholesterol levels and increase the risk of heart disease, so it's best to limit intake as much as possible.

2. Healthy Fat Choices:

- **Sources of Monounsaturated Fats:** Include olive oil, avocado oil, avocados, nuts (e.g., almonds, cashews, peanuts), and seeds (e.g., pumpkin seeds, sesame seeds).

- **Sources of Polyunsaturated Fats:** Include fatty fish (e.g., salmon, trout, mackerel), flaxseeds, chia seeds, walnuts, soybeans, and tofu. Aim to consume a variety of omega-3 and omega-6 sources for optimal health.

- **Limit Saturated and Trans Fats:** Choose lean cuts of meat, poultry without skin, low-fat dairy products, and limit consumption of processed meats and high-fat dairy. Avoid foods containing partially hydrogenated oils and minimize intake of fried foods, baked goods, and snacks with trans fats.

- **Healthy Cooking Methods:** Opt for cooking methods that use minimal added fats, such as grilling, baking, broiling, steaming, or sautéing with small amounts of olive oil or avocado oil.

- **Read Food Labels:** Check food labels for the types and amounts of fats in packaged foods. Choose products with lower saturated and trans fat content and prioritize foods with healthier fat sources.

3. Balance and Moderation:
  - While it's essential to choose healthier fats, it's also important to consume fats in moderation as part of a balanced diet. Aim to incorporate a variety of healthy fats into your meals and snacks while staying within your recommended daily calorie intake.
  - Remember that fats are calorie-dense, so be mindful of portion sizes and avoid excessive consumption, even of healthy fats.

The Importance of Fiber in the Diet

Fiber is an essential component of a healthy diet and plays numerous important roles in promoting overall health and well-being. Understanding the importance of fiber in the diet is crucial for making informed dietary choices. Here's why fiber is essential:

1. Digestive Health:
  - Fiber promotes digestive health by adding bulk to stools and supporting regular bowel movements. It helps prevent constipation by softening stools and easing their passage through the digestive tract.
  - Additionally, fiber can help alleviate symptoms of diarrhea by absorbing excess water and promoting firmer stools.

2. Weight Management:
  - High-fiber foods tend to be more filling and satisfying than low-fiber foods, which can help control appetite and reduce calorie intake.
  - Including fiber-rich foods in meals and snacks can promote satiety, prevent overeating, and support weight management efforts by reducing overall calorie consumption.

3. Blood Sugar Control:
  - Fiber plays a crucial role in regulating blood sugar levels by slowing the absorption of glucose from the digestive tract into the bloodstream.
  - Soluble fiber, found in foods like oats, beans, and fruits, forms a gel-like substance in the digestive tract that helps stabilize blood sugar levels and prevent spikes and crashes.

4. Heart Health:

- High-fiber diets are associated with a reduced risk of heart disease and stroke. Soluble fiber helps lower LDL (bad) cholesterol levels by binding to cholesterol particles in the digestive tract and removing them from the body.
- Additionally, fiber-rich foods can help lower blood pressure, improve blood vessel function, and reduce inflammation, all of which contribute to heart health.

5. Gut Microbiome Health:

- Fiber serves as a prebiotic, feeding beneficial bacteria in the gut and promoting a healthy balance of gut microbiota.
- A diverse and thriving gut microbiome is associated with improved digestion, immune function, metabolism, and mental health.

6. Reduced Risk of Chronic Diseases:

- High-fiber diets are linked to a lower risk of chronic diseases such as type 2 diabetes, certain cancers (e.g., colorectal cancer), and digestive disorders (e.g., diverticulitis).
- Fiber-rich foods provide essential nutrients, antioxidants, and phytochemicals that support overall health and reduce inflammation and oxidative stress in the body.

7. Sources of Fiber:

- Fiber is found in plant-based foods such as fruits, vegetables, whole grains, legumes, nuts, and seeds.
- Examples of high-fiber foods include berries, apples, oranges, broccoli, spinach, carrots, whole grains (e.g., oats, brown rice, quinoa), beans, lentils, chickpeas, almonds, chia seeds, and flaxseeds.

8. Recommended Intake:

- The Dietary Guidelines for Americans recommend consuming a variety of fiber-rich foods and aiming for a daily intake of 25 grams for women and 38 grams for men, although individual needs may vary.
- Gradually increase fiber intake and drink plenty of water to prevent digestive discomfort and bloating associated with sudden dietary changes.

Balancing Macronutrients for Optimal Health

Balancing macronutrients—carbohydrates, proteins, and fats—in your diet is essential for optimal health and well-being. Each macronutrient serves a unique role in the body, and finding the right balance can support various aspects of health, including energy levels, metabolism, muscle growth, and overall vitality. Here's how to balance macronutrients for optimal health:

1. Understand Your Nutrient Needs:
   - Start by understanding your individual nutrient needs based on factors such as age, sex, weight, height, activity level, and health goals. Consider consulting with a registered dietitian or nutritionist for personalized guidance.

2. Prioritize Whole Foods:
   - Focus on consuming a variety of whole, nutrient-dense foods that provide a balance of macronutrients, vitamins, minerals, and antioxidants. Choose minimally processed foods over highly processed and refined options whenever possible.

3. Emphasize High-Quality Carbohydrates:
   - Choose complex carbohydrates from whole grains, fruits, vegetables, legumes, and starchy vegetables as the foundation of your diet. Aim to include a variety of colorful fruits and vegetables in your meals to maximize nutrient intake and fiber content.

4. Include Lean Proteins:
   - Incorporate lean protein sources such as poultry, fish, eggs, tofu, tempeh, legumes, and low-fat dairy products into your meals and snacks. Protein helps support muscle growth, repair, and satiety, so aim to include a source of protein in each meal.

5. Opt for Healthy Fats:
   - Choose healthy fats from sources such as olive oil, avocados, nuts, seeds, fatty fish, and plant-based oils. Limit saturated fats from animal products and processed foods, and avoid trans fats altogether.

6. Balance Portion Sizes:

- Pay attention to portion sizes and aim to balance macronutrients in each meal and snack. Include a combination of carbohydrates, proteins, and fats to provide sustained energy, promote satiety, and support overall nutrition.

7. Consider Your Activity Level:

- Adjust your macronutrient intake based on your activity level and fitness goals. Active individuals may need slightly higher protein intake to support muscle repair and recovery, while endurance athletes may benefit from higher carbohydrate intake to fuel performance.

8. Listen to Your Body:

- Pay attention to hunger and fullness cues, and eat mindfully to avoid overeating or undereating. Experiment with different macronutrient ratios and meal timings to find what works best for your body and lifestyle.

9. Stay Hydrated:

- Don't forget about hydration! Water is essential for overall health and helps regulate appetite, digestion, and metabolism. Aim to drink plenty of water throughout the day, especially before and after exercise.

10. Be Flexible and Enjoy Food:

- While it's essential to strive for balance and moderation, remember that no single meal or food choice will make or break your health. Allow yourself flexibility and enjoy a variety of foods in moderation, including occasional treats or indulgences.

Chapter 5
Micronutrients and Their Functions

Vitamins: Sources and Functions

Vitamins are essential micronutrients that play crucial roles in various physiological functions, including metabolism, immune function, and cell repair. Each vitamin has unique functions and dietary sources. Here's an overview of vitamins, their sources, and functions:

1. Vitamin A:
  - **Sources:** Found in foods such as liver, fish oils, dairy products, eggs, and orange and yellow fruits and vegetables (e.g., carrots, sweet potatoes, pumpkins, apricots, mangoes).
  - **Functions:** Essential for vision health, immune function, skin health, and cell growth and differentiation. Also important for reproductive health and fetal development.

2. Vitamin B Complex:
  - **Sources:** Various foods, including whole grains, fortified cereals, meat, poultry, fish, eggs, dairy products, legumes, leafy green vegetables, nuts, and seeds.
  - **Functions:** The B-complex vitamins include thiamine (B1), riboflavin (B2), niacin (B3), pantothenic acid (B5), pyridoxine (B6), biotin (B7), folate (B9), and cobalamin (B12). They play key roles in energy metabolism, nerve function, red blood cell formation, DNA synthesis, and neurotransmitter production.

3. Vitamin C:
  - **Sources:** Found in citrus fruits (e.g., oranges, lemons), berries, kiwi, tomatoes, peppers (e.g., red bell peppers), broccoli, Brussels sprouts, and leafy green vegetables.
  - **Functions:** Acts as an antioxidant, protecting cells from damage caused by free radicals. Essential for collagen synthesis, wound healing, immune function, and iron absorption.

4. Vitamin D:
  - **Sources:** Mainly obtained through sunlight exposure, as well as some foods such as fatty fish (e.g., salmon, mackerel), fortified dairy and plant-based milk, egg yolks, and liver.

- **Functions:** Critical for bone health and calcium metabolism, as it helps regulate calcium and phosphate absorption in the intestines. Also plays a role in immune function and may have other health benefits.

5. Vitamin E:
- **Sources:** Found in nuts, seeds, vegetable oils (e.g., sunflower oil, safflower oil, almond oil), leafy green vegetables, avocados, and fortified cereals.
- **Functions:** Acts as an antioxidant, protecting cell membranes from oxidative damage. Important for immune function, skin health, and neurological function.

6. Vitamin K:
- **Sources:** Found in leafy green vegetables (e.g., spinach, kale, Swiss chard), broccoli, Brussels sprouts, cabbage, and certain vegetable oils (e.g., soybean oil, canola oil).
- **Functions:** Essential for blood clotting, as it helps activate proteins involved in the coagulation process. Also plays a role in bone metabolism and may have other functions.

7. Vitamin B12:
- **Sources:** Found almost exclusively in animal products such as meat, poultry, fish, eggs, and dairy. Fortified foods and supplements are available for vegetarians and vegans.
- **Functions:** Essential for red blood cell formation, neurological function, and DNA synthesis. Plays a critical role in nerve health and may help prevent certain types of anemia.

8. Vitamin B9 (Folate):
- **Sources:** Found in leafy green vegetables, legumes, citrus fruits, fortified cereals, and liver. Folic acid is the synthetic form found in supplements and fortified foods.
- **Functions:** Important for DNA synthesis, cell division, and red blood cell formation. Essential for fetal development during pregnancy and may help prevent neural tube defects.

Minerals: Essential for Health

Minerals are essential micronutrients that play critical roles in various physiological functions, including bone health, muscle function, fluid balance, and nerve transmission. Here's an overview of minerals and their importance for health:

1. Calcium:
  - **Functions:** Essential for bone and teeth health, muscle contraction, nerve transmission, and blood clotting.
  - **Sources:** Dairy products (e.g., milk, yogurt, cheese), leafy green vegetables (e.g., kale, spinach), fortified plant-based milk, tofu, almonds, and calcium-fortified foods.

2. Iron:
  - **Functions:** Necessary for oxygen transport in the blood, energy metabolism, and immune function.
  - **Sources:** Red meat, poultry, fish, beans, lentils, tofu, fortified cereals, spinach, and other leafy green vegetables.

3. Magnesium:
  - **Functions:** Supports muscle and nerve function, energy metabolism, bone health, and blood pressure regulation.
  - **Sources:** Nuts (e.g., almonds, cashews), seeds (e.g., pumpkin seeds, sunflower seeds), whole grains (e.g., brown rice, oats, quinoa), leafy green vegetables, and legumes.

4. Potassium:
  - **Functions:** Helps maintain fluid balance, nerve function, muscle contractions, and blood pressure regulation.
  - **Sources:** Bananas, oranges, potatoes, sweet potatoes, tomatoes, spinach, beans, yogurt, and fish.

5. Sodium:
  - **Functions:** Necessary for fluid balance, nerve transmission, and muscle function. However, excessive sodium intake can lead to high blood pressure and other health issues.
  - **Sources:** Table salt, processed and packaged foods, canned soups, sauces, and snacks.

6. Zinc:

- **Functions:** Supports immune function, wound healing, DNA synthesis, and growth and development.
  - **Sources:** Oysters, red meat, poultry, beans, nuts, seeds, whole grains, and dairy products.

7. Phosphorus:
  - **Functions:** Important for bone and teeth health, energy metabolism, and cell structure.
  - **Sources:** Meat, poultry, fish, dairy products, nuts, seeds, beans, and whole grains.

8. Iodine:
  - **Functions:** Essential for thyroid function and the production of thyroid hormones, which regulate metabolism.
  - **Sources:** Seafood (e.g., fish, seaweed), dairy products, iodized salt, and some fruits and vegetables grown in iodine-rich soil.

9. Selenium:
  - **Functions:** Acts as an antioxidant, supports thyroid function, and helps regulate immune function.
  - **Sources:** Brazil nuts, seafood, poultry, eggs, whole grains, and dairy products.

10. Copper:
  - **Functions:** Necessary for energy production, iron metabolism, and the formation of connective tissues.
  - **Sources:** Shellfish, nuts, seeds, whole grains, beans, and organ meats.

11. Manganese:
  - **Functions:** Supports bone health, carbohydrate metabolism, and antioxidant defense.
  - **Sources:** Nuts, seeds, whole grains, leafy green vegetables, tea, and pineapple.

12. Chromium:
  - **Functions:** Helps regulate blood sugar levels by enhancing the action of insulin.
  - **Sources:** Broccoli, whole grains, nuts, seeds, and brewer's yeast.

13. Molybdenum:
   - **Functions:** Assists in the metabolism of certain amino acids and the detoxification of sulfites.
   - **Sources:** Legumes, grains, nuts, leafy green vegetables, and organ meats.

14. Fluoride:
   - **Functions:** Supports dental health by strengthening tooth enamel and preventing tooth decay.
   - **Sources:** Fluoridated water, tea, seafood, and some toothpaste and dental products.

Antioxidants and Their Role in Disease Prevention

Antioxidants are compounds that help neutralize harmful molecules called free radicals, which can damage cells and contribute to various diseases and aging processes. Consuming foods rich in antioxidants can help protect against oxidative stress and reduce the risk of chronic diseases. Here's how antioxidants play a crucial role in disease prevention:

1. Neutralizing Free Radicals:
   - Free radicals are unstable molecules with unpaired electrons, which can cause oxidative damage to cells, DNA, proteins, and lipids.
   - Antioxidants donate electrons to stabilize free radicals, preventing them from causing further damage and reducing oxidative stress in the body.

2. Protecting Against Chronic Diseases:
   - Oxidative stress is associated with the development of chronic diseases such as heart disease, cancer, diabetes, neurodegenerative disorders (e.g., Alzheimer's disease, Parkinson's disease), and inflammatory conditions.
   - Antioxidants help reduce inflammation, protect against DNA damage, and inhibit the growth of cancer cells, thus lowering the risk of chronic diseases.

3. Supporting Heart Health:

- Antioxidants such as vitamins C and E, flavonoids, and polyphenols help protect against cardiovascular disease by reducing oxidative damage to blood vessels, lowering inflammation, and improving blood vessel function.
- Consuming a diet rich in antioxidant-rich foods is associated with a lower risk of heart disease and stroke.

4. Enhancing Immune Function:

- Antioxidants play a crucial role in supporting immune function by protecting immune cells from oxidative damage and inflammation.
- Vitamins A, C, and E, along with minerals like selenium and zinc, help strengthen the immune system and improve resistance to infections and illness.

5. Supporting Brain Health:

- Oxidative stress and inflammation are implicated in the development of neurodegenerative diseases such as Alzheimer's and Parkinson's disease.
- Antioxidants, particularly flavonoids and polyphenols found in fruits, vegetables, and tea, may help protect against cognitive decline, improve memory, and reduce the risk of neurodegenerative disorders.

6. Protecting Against Aging:

- Oxidative stress contributes to the aging process by damaging cells and tissues, leading to wrinkles, age spots, and reduced organ function.
- Antioxidants help counteract oxidative damage and protect against premature aging by maintaining cellular integrity and function.

7. Dietary Sources of Antioxidants:

- Antioxidants are found in a wide variety of foods, particularly plant-based foods such as fruits, vegetables, nuts, seeds, whole grains, herbs, and spices.
- Examples of antioxidant-rich foods include berries (e.g., blueberries, strawberries, raspberries), citrus fruits, leafy green vegetables, tomatoes, carrots, sweet potatoes, nuts (e.g., almonds, walnuts), seeds (e.g., flaxseeds, chia seeds), green tea, and dark chocolate.

Trace Elements and Micronutrient Balance

Trace elements, also known as trace minerals or microminerals, are essential nutrients required by the body in smaller amounts compared to macronutrients like carbohydrates, proteins, and fats. Despite their small quantities, these trace elements play crucial roles in various physiological functions and overall health. Maintaining a proper balance of micronutrients is essential for optimal health. Here's an overview of some important trace elements and their functions, along with the importance of micronutrient balance:

1. Iron:
  - **Function:** Iron is essential for oxygen transport in the blood as a component of hemoglobin and myoglobin. It also plays a role in energy metabolism.
  - **Sources:** Red meat, poultry, fish, beans, lentils, tofu, fortified cereals, spinach, and other leafy green vegetables.
  - **Importance of Balance:** Iron deficiency can lead to anemia and impaired oxygen delivery to tissues, while excessive iron intake can cause toxicity and oxidative damage.

2. Zinc:
  - **Function:** Zinc is involved in immune function, wound healing, DNA synthesis, growth and development, and taste perception.
  - **Sources:** Oysters, red meat, poultry, beans, nuts, seeds, dairy products, and whole grains.
  - **Importance of Balance:** Zinc deficiency can impair immune function and wound healing, while excessive zinc intake can interfere with copper absorption and cause toxicity symptoms.

3. Copper:
  - **Function:** Copper is essential for the formation of red blood cells, connective tissues, and enzymes involved in energy metabolism and antioxidant defense.
  - **Sources:** Shellfish, nuts, seeds, beans, whole grains, organ meats, and cocoa.
  - **Importance of Balance:** Copper deficiency can lead to anemia, impaired immune function, and connective tissue disorders, while excessive copper intake can cause toxicity and liver damage.

4. Selenium:

- **Function:** Selenium acts as an antioxidant, supporting immune function, thyroid health, and DNA synthesis.
- **Sources:** Brazil nuts, seafood (e.g., fish, shellfish), poultry, eggs, dairy products, and whole grains.
- **Importance of Balance:** Selenium deficiency is associated with an increased risk of certain cancers and thyroid disorders, while excessive selenium intake can lead to toxicity and selenosis.

5. Iodine:

- **Function:** Iodine is essential for thyroid hormone synthesis, which regulates metabolism, growth, and development.
- **Sources:** Seafood (e.g., fish, seaweed), dairy products, iodized salt, and some fruits and vegetables grown in iodine-rich soil.
- **Importance of Balance:** Iodine deficiency can lead to hypothyroidism and goiter, while excessive iodine intake can disrupt thyroid function and cause thyroid disorders.

6. Manganese:

- **Function:** Manganese is involved in bone formation, carbohydrate metabolism, antioxidant defense, and enzyme activation.
- **Sources:** Nuts, seeds, whole grains, leafy green vegetables, tea, and pineapple.
- **Importance of Balance:** Manganese deficiency is rare but can impair growth and bone health, while excessive manganese intake can cause neurological symptoms and toxicity.

7. Fluoride:

- **Function:** Fluoride helps strengthen tooth enamel and prevent tooth decay by promoting remineralization and inhibiting bacterial growth.
- **Sources:** Fluoridated water, tea, seafood, and some toothpaste and dental products.
- **Importance of Balance:** Fluoride intake should be balanced to prevent dental fluorosis (excessive fluoride intake during tooth development) without compromising dental health.

8. Chromium:

  - **Function:** Chromium helps regulate blood sugar levels by enhancing insulin sensitivity and glucose uptake into cells.
  - **Sources:** Broccoli, whole grains, nuts, seeds, and brewer's yeast.
  - **Importance of Balance:** Chromium deficiency can impair glucose metabolism and increase the risk of insulin resistance, while excessive chromium intake may have adverse effects on renal function.

Maintaining a proper balance of trace elements is crucial for overall health and well-being. While these micronutrients are required in small amounts, their functions are vital for various physiological processes. Consuming a diverse and balanced diet rich in whole foods can help ensure adequate intake of trace elements and support optimal health. If needed, dietary supplements may be used to fill nutrient gaps, but it's important to avoid excessive intake and strive for balance to prevent nutrient imbalances and potential adverse effects.

Meeting Micronutrient Needs Through Diet

Meeting micronutrient needs through diet is essential for overall health and well-being. Micronutrients, including vitamins and minerals, play crucial roles in various physiological functions, such as immune function, metabolism, bone health, and energy production. Here's how to ensure you're meeting your micronutrient needs through your diet:

1. Eat a Variety of Nutrient-Dense Foods:
  - Consume a diverse range of whole foods, including fruits, vegetables, whole grains, lean proteins, dairy or dairy alternatives, nuts, seeds, and legumes.
  - Aim to include a variety of colors in your meals, as different colored fruits and vegetables contain unique combinations of vitamins, minerals, and antioxidants.

2. Prioritize Fruits and Vegetables:
  - Aim to fill half your plate with fruits and vegetables at each meal. Choose a variety of colors, as different colors indicate different phytonutrients and micronutrient profiles.

- Include both raw and cooked vegetables in your diet to maximize nutrient intake. Steaming or lightly cooking vegetables helps retain their nutritional value.

3. Include Lean Proteins:
- Incorporate lean sources of protein into your meals, such as poultry, fish, seafood, tofu, tempeh, legumes, beans, lentils, and low-fat dairy products.
- Protein-rich foods provide essential amino acids and micronutrients like iron, zinc, and B vitamins, which are important for muscle repair, immune function, and overall health.

4. Choose Whole Grains:
- Opt for whole grains such as brown rice, quinoa, oats, barley, whole wheat bread, and whole grain pasta instead of refined grains.
- Whole grains are rich in vitamins (e.g., B vitamins) and minerals (e.g., magnesium, selenium) and provide fiber for digestive health and satiety.

5. Include Healthy Fats:
- Incorporate sources of healthy fats into your diet, such as avocados, nuts, seeds, olive oil, fatty fish (e.g., salmon, mackerel), and coconut oil (in moderation).
- Healthy fats are important for absorption of fat-soluble vitamins (A, D, E, K) and provide essential fatty acids like omega-3 and omega-6, which support brain health and inflammation regulation.

6. Consume Dairy or Dairy Alternatives:
- Include dairy products or fortified dairy alternatives in your diet to meet calcium and vitamin D needs for bone health.
- Choose low-fat or non-fat dairy options to reduce saturated fat intake while still obtaining essential nutrients like calcium, vitamin D, and protein.

7. Limit Processed and Sugary Foods:
- Minimize consumption of processed and sugary foods, as they often provide empty calories and lack essential micronutrients.
- Instead, focus on nutrient-dense whole foods that provide a wide range of vitamins, minerals, and other beneficial compounds.

8. Read Food Labels:
   - Pay attention to food labels to identify nutrient-rich foods and make informed choices about your diet.
   - Look for foods that are rich in vitamins, minerals, and other beneficial nutrients while being mindful of added sugars, sodium, and unhealthy fats.

9. Consider Supplementation if Necessary:
   - If you have specific dietary restrictions, food allergies, or medical conditions that may impact nutrient absorption, consult with a healthcare provider or registered dietitian to determine if supplementation is necessary.
   - Supplements should complement a balanced diet and should not be used as a substitute for nutrient-rich foods.

Chapter 6
Healthy Eating Patterns

Mediterranean Diet: A Model for Health

The Mediterranean diet is widely recognized as one of the healthiest eating patterns, supported by extensive research demonstrating its numerous health benefits. This dietary model is inspired by the traditional eating habits of people living in countries bordering the Mediterranean Sea, such as Greece, Italy, Spain, and southern France. Here's an overview of the Mediterranean diet and why it's considered a model for health:

1. Emphasis on Plant-Based Foods:
   - The Mediterranean diet is predominantly plant-based, with a focus on fruits, vegetables, whole grains, legumes, nuts, seeds, and olive oil.
   - These foods are rich in vitamins, minerals, antioxidants, fiber, and phytonutrients, which support overall health and reduce the risk of chronic diseases.

2. Olive Oil as the Primary Fat:
   - Olive oil is the primary source of fat in the Mediterranean diet and is used for cooking, salad dressings, and dips.
   - Rich in monounsaturated fats and antioxidants, olive oil is associated with a reduced risk of heart disease, inflammation, and oxidative stress.

3. Moderate Consumption of Fish and Poultry:
   - The Mediterranean diet includes moderate amounts of fish and poultry, with an emphasis on fatty fish such as salmon, mackerel, sardines, and trout.
   - Fish is a rich source of omega-3 fatty acids, which are beneficial for heart health, brain function, and inflammation regulation.

4. Limited Red Meat Intake:
   - Red meat consumption is limited in the Mediterranean diet, with a focus on leaner protein sources like poultry, fish, and plant-based proteins.
   - This dietary pattern reduces intake of saturated fats and cholesterol, which are associated with an increased risk of heart disease and other chronic conditions.

5. Regular Consumption of Dairy Products:
   - The Mediterranean diet includes moderate amounts of dairy products, such as yogurt, cheese, and milk.
   - These foods provide calcium, protein, and other essential nutrients important for bone health and overall well-being.

6. Emphasis on Herbs and Spices:
   - Herbs and spices are used liberally in Mediterranean cuisine to add flavor and aroma to dishes without relying on excess salt or added sugars.
   - Common herbs and spices include basil, oregano, thyme, rosemary, garlic, and cinnamon, which offer both culinary and health benefits.

7. Daily Consumption of Fruits and Vegetables:
   - Fruits and vegetables are staple foods in the Mediterranean diet, consumed in abundance at every meal.
   - These foods are rich in vitamins, minerals, antioxidants, and fiber, which promote digestive health, immune function, and disease prevention.

8. Moderate Consumption of Wine:
   - Moderate consumption of red wine, typically consumed with meals, is a characteristic feature of the Mediterranean diet.
   - Red wine contains antioxidants like resveratrol, which may have protective effects against heart disease and inflammation. However, it's important to consume alcohol in moderation and avoid excessive intake.

9. Social and Lifestyle Factors:
   - The Mediterranean diet is not just about food but also incorporates social and lifestyle factors, such as enjoying meals with family and friends, being physically active, and engaging in regular exercise.
   - These aspects of the Mediterranean lifestyle contribute to overall health and well-being, reducing stress and promoting mental and emotional health.

10. Health Benefits:

- Numerous studies have shown that adherence to the Mediterranean diet is associated with a reduced risk of heart disease, stroke, type 2 diabetes, certain cancers, Alzheimer's disease, and overall mortality.
- The combination of nutrient-rich foods, healthy fats, antioxidants, and lifestyle factors in the Mediterranean diet supports longevity and vitality.

DASH Diet: Promoting Heart Health

The DASH (Dietary Approaches to Stop Hypertension) diet is a dietary pattern designed to promote heart health and lower blood pressure. Developed by the National Institutes of Health (NIH), the DASH diet emphasizes nutrient-rich foods and limits sodium intake. Here's an overview of the DASH diet and its principles for promoting heart health:

1. Emphasis on Fruits and Vegetables:
- The DASH diet encourages the consumption of fruits and vegetables, which are rich in vitamins, minerals, antioxidants, and fiber.
- Aim to include a variety of colorful fruits and vegetables in your meals and snacks to maximize nutrient intake and support heart health.

2. Whole Grains as the Main Source of Carbohydrates:
- Whole grains provide complex carbohydrates, fiber, and essential nutrients. They are a key component of the DASH diet.
- Choose whole grain options such as brown rice, quinoa, whole wheat bread, oats, barley, and whole grain pasta over refined grains.

3. Lean Protein Sources:
- The DASH diet includes lean protein sources such as poultry, fish, seafood, beans, lentils, tofu, and low-fat dairy products.
- Limit intake of red meat and opt for leaner protein options to reduce saturated fat intake and support heart health.

4. Healthy Fats:
- Healthy fats, such as those found in nuts, seeds, avocados, and olive oil, are emphasized in the DASH diet.

- These fats provide essential fatty acids and antioxidants, which help reduce inflammation and support cardiovascular health.

5. Low-Fat Dairy Products:

- Low-fat or non-fat dairy products are recommended in the DASH diet to lower intake of saturated fat and cholesterol.
- Choose options like skim milk, low-fat yogurt, and reduced-fat cheese to support heart health while still obtaining essential nutrients like calcium and vitamin D.

6. Limited Sodium Intake:

- The DASH diet restricts sodium intake to help lower blood pressure and reduce the risk of hypertension and heart disease.
- Aim to consume no more than 2,300 milligrams of sodium per day, and ideally, aim for 1,500 milligrams per day for even greater blood pressure reduction.

7. Moderation with Added Sugars and Sweets:

- While the DASH diet doesn't eliminate sweets entirely, it encourages moderation and mindful consumption of added sugars and sugary foods.
- Limit intake of sugary beverages, desserts, and processed foods high in added sugars to support overall health and weight management.

8. Portion Control and Balanced Meals:

- Pay attention to portion sizes and aim for balanced meals that include a variety of nutrient-rich foods from all food groups.
- Focus on filling half your plate with fruits and vegetables, one-quarter with lean protein, and one-quarter with whole grains or starchy vegetables.

9. Regular Physical Activity:

- Along with following the DASH diet, regular physical activity is recommended to further support heart health and overall well-being.
- Aim for at least 150 minutes of moderate-intensity aerobic exercise or 75 minutes of vigorous-intensity exercise per week, along with muscle-strengthening activities on two or more days per week.

10. Benefits for Heart Health:

- Numerous studies have shown that adherence to the DASH diet is associated with lower blood pressure, reduced risk of hypertension, and improved cardiovascular health.
- The combination of nutrient-rich foods, limited sodium intake, and lifestyle factors in the DASH diet supports heart health and may help prevent heart disease and stroke.

Plant-Based Diets: Benefits and Considerations

Plant-based diets emphasize foods derived from plants, including fruits, vegetables, whole grains, nuts, seeds, and legumes, while minimizing or excluding animal products. These diets have gained popularity due to their numerous health benefits and positive environmental impact. Here's an overview of the benefits and considerations of plant-based diets:

Benefits:

1. **Rich in Nutrients:** Plant-based diets are naturally high in vitamins, minerals, antioxidants, and phytonutrients found in fruits, vegetables, whole grains, nuts, and seeds. These nutrients support overall health and reduce the risk of chronic diseases.

2. **Lower Risk of Chronic Diseases:** Research shows that plant-based diets are associated with a reduced risk of heart disease, high blood pressure, type 2 diabetes, certain cancers, and obesity. These diets are typically lower in saturated fat and cholesterol and higher in fiber and beneficial plant compounds, which contribute to better health outcomes.

3. **Weight Management:** Plant-based diets are often lower in calorie density and higher in fiber, which can promote feelings of fullness and satiety, leading to weight loss or weight maintenance. Research suggests that individuals following plant-based diets tend to have lower body weight and body mass index (BMI).

4. **Improved Digestive Health:** The high fiber content of plant-based diets promotes digestive health by supporting regular bowel

movements, preventing constipation, and reducing the risk of
gastrointestinal disorders such as diverticulosis and hemorrhoids.

5. **Environmental Sustainability:** Plant-based diets have a lower
environmental footprint compared to diets high in animal products.
Producing plant foods requires fewer natural resources, produces fewer
greenhouse gas emissions, and uses less land and water, making plant-
based diets more sustainable and environmentally friendly.

6. **Ethical Considerations:** Many people choose plant-based diets for
ethical reasons, including concerns about animal welfare and the
environmental impact of animal agriculture. Plant-based diets promote
compassion towards animals and support more sustainable and humane
food production practices.

Considerations:

1. **Nutrient Considerations:** While plant-based diets can provide
adequate nutrition when well-planned, it's important to pay attention
to certain nutrients that may be lacking, such as vitamin B12, vitamin
D, omega-3 fatty acids, iron, calcium, zinc, and protein. Consider
incorporating fortified foods or supplements to ensure adequate intake
of these nutrients.

2. **Protein Quality:** Plant-based sources of protein may not always
provide all essential amino acids in optimal proportions. However,
consuming a variety of protein-rich plant foods such as legumes, tofu,
tempeh, seitan, nuts, seeds, and grains throughout the day can ensure
adequate protein intake and amino acid balance.

3. **Meal Planning:** Planning balanced meals and snacks that include a
variety of plant foods is essential for meeting nutrient needs on a
plant-based diet. Focus on incorporating a rainbow of colorful fruits
and vegetables, whole grains, plant-based proteins, healthy fats, and
fortified foods into your meals.

4. **Social and Practical Considerations:** Following a plant-based diet
may require adjustments in social situations, dining out, and meal
preparation. It's important to communicate your dietary preferences

and needs with friends, family, and restaurants to ensure you have access to plant-based options that align with your lifestyle.

5. **Individual Variation:** Plant-based diets can vary widely in their composition, ranging from vegan diets that exclude all animal products to vegetarian diets that may include dairy and eggs. Choose the type of plant-based diet that best suits your personal preferences, cultural background, nutritional needs, and health goals.

The Role of Mindful Eating

Mindful eating is a practice that encourages awareness and presence during meals, allowing individuals to fully engage with their food and eating experience. It involves paying attention to the sensory aspects of eating, such as taste, texture, smell, and sight, as well as recognizing hunger and satiety cues. Here's an overview of the role of mindful eating in promoting healthy eating patterns:

1. Increased Awareness:
  - Mindful eating cultivates a heightened awareness of the eating experience, including the physical sensations, thoughts, and emotions associated with food and eating.
  - By being present in the moment, individuals can develop a deeper understanding of their dietary habits, preferences, and relationship with food.

2. Recognition of Hunger and Fullness:
  - Mindful eating helps individuals tune into their body's hunger and satiety cues, allowing them to distinguish between physical hunger and other triggers for eating, such as emotions or external cues.
  - By eating when hungry and stopping when satisfied, mindful eaters can better regulate their food intake and avoid overeating or undereating.

3. Prevention of Emotional Eating:
  - Mindful eating encourages nonjudgmental awareness of emotions and urges related to food and eating.

- By recognizing and acknowledging emotional triggers for eating, individuals can develop healthier coping mechanisms and respond to emotional cues without turning to food for comfort or distraction.

4. Enhanced Enjoyment of Food:
- Mindful eating promotes a greater appreciation and enjoyment of food by focusing on the sensory experience of eating.
- By savoring each bite and paying attention to flavors, textures, and aromas, individuals can derive more satisfaction from their meals and snacks, leading to greater culinary pleasure and fulfillment.

5. Improved Digestion and Nutrient Absorption:
- Eating mindfully involves chewing food slowly and thoroughly, which aids in digestion and nutrient absorption.
- By taking the time to chew food properly, individuals can promote better digestion, reduce digestive discomfort, and optimize the body's utilization of nutrients from food.

6. Reduction of Mindless Eating Behaviors:
- Mindful eating helps individuals become more conscious of habitual or automatic eating behaviors, such as eating in front of the TV, eating out of boredom, or snacking without awareness.
- By bringing awareness to these behaviors, individuals can make more intentional choices about when, what, and how much they eat, leading to healthier eating patterns and improved food satisfaction.

7. Stress Reduction and Mind-Body Connection:
- Mindful eating encourages relaxation and stress reduction through focused attention on the present moment and the act of eating.
- By practicing mindfulness techniques during meals, such as deep breathing or body scanning, individuals can cultivate a greater sense of calmness, resilience, and connection to their body's needs.

8. Promotion of Intuitive Eating:
- Mindful eating aligns with the principles of intuitive eating, which emphasizes listening to the body's hunger and fullness cues, rejecting diet mentality, and honoring physical and emotional well-being.
- By integrating mindfulness into eating habits, individuals can develop a more intuitive and balanced approach to food and

nourishment, free from restrictive dieting and food-related guilt or shame.

Customizing Dietary Patterns for Individual Needs

Customizing dietary patterns for individual needs involves tailoring dietary choices and eating habits to meet specific health goals, preferences, cultural practices, and lifestyle factors. Here's an overview of how to customize dietary patterns for individual needs:

1. Assessing Nutritional Needs:
 - Start by assessing your individual nutritional needs based on factors such as age, sex, weight, height, activity level, health status, and any specific dietary requirements or restrictions.
 - Consider consulting with a registered dietitian or healthcare provider to determine your unique nutritional needs and develop a personalized eating plan.

2. Setting Health Goals:
 - Identify specific health goals or objectives you want to achieve through your diet, such as improving heart health, managing weight, supporting athletic performance, managing chronic conditions (e.g., diabetes, hypertension), or addressing food allergies or intolerances.
 - Set realistic and achievable goals that are aligned with your health priorities and lifestyle.

3. Consider Cultural and Personal Preferences:
 - Take into account cultural and personal food preferences, traditions, and dietary habits when customizing your eating pattern.
 - Incorporate familiar and culturally relevant foods into your meals while making modifications to improve nutritional quality and support your health goals.

4. Adapting Dietary Patterns:
 - Choose a dietary pattern or approach that aligns with your health goals and preferences, such as the Mediterranean diet, DASH diet, plant-based diet, low-carb diet, or ketogenic diet.

- Modify and adapt the chosen dietary pattern to suit your individual needs and preferences, making adjustments as needed to meet nutritional requirements and lifestyle factors.

5. Tailoring Macronutrient Intake:
- Customize your macronutrient intake (carbohydrates, proteins, and fats) based on your energy needs, activity level, metabolic health, and personal preferences.
- Experiment with different macronutrient ratios to find the balance that works best for you in terms of energy levels, satiety, and overall well-being.

6. Addressing Nutrient Deficiencies:
- Identify and address any nutrient deficiencies or imbalances in your diet by incorporating nutrient-rich foods and, if necessary, considering dietary supplements under the guidance of a healthcare professional.
- Focus on including a variety of nutrient-dense foods from all food groups to ensure you're meeting your daily nutrient needs.

7. Listening to Your Body:
- Practice intuitive eating by listening to your body's hunger and fullness cues, as well as cravings and preferences, to guide your food choices and eating habits.
- Tune in to how different foods make you feel physically, mentally, and emotionally, and adjust your diet accordingly to support overall well-being.

8. Being Flexible and Adaptable:
- Remain flexible and adaptable with your dietary patterns, recognizing that nutritional needs may change over time due to factors such as age, life stage, physical activity, and health status.
- Be open to making adjustments to your diet as needed to accommodate changing circumstances and optimize your health and well-being.

9. Seeking Professional Guidance:
- If you're unsure about how to customize your dietary patterns or have specific health concerns or conditions, seek guidance from a

registered dietitian or healthcare provider who can provide personalized nutrition advice and support.

  - Work collaboratively with a nutrition professional to develop a customized eating plan that meets your individual needs, preferences, and health goals.

Chapter 7
Meal Planning and Preparation

The Importance of Meal Planning

Meal planning is a key component of healthy eating habits and can have numerous benefits for individuals looking to improve their nutrition and overall well-being. Here's an overview of the importance of meal planning:

1. Promotes Nutritional Balance:
  - Meal planning allows you to create balanced meals that include a variety of nutrient-rich foods from all food groups, such as fruits, vegetables, whole grains, lean proteins, and healthy fats.
  - By carefully selecting ingredients and recipes in advance, you can ensure that your meals provide essential vitamins, minerals, antioxidants, and macronutrients needed for optimal health.

2. Supports Health Goals:
  - Meal planning helps individuals align their eating habits with their health goals, whether they're aiming to lose weight, improve athletic performance, manage chronic conditions, or simply adopt a healthier lifestyle.
  - By setting specific goals and planning meals accordingly, you can make intentional food choices that support your desired outcomes and long-term health objectives.

3. Saves Time and Money:
  - Planning meals in advance can save time and money by reducing the need for frequent grocery store trips, last-minute meal decisions, and dining out.
  - With a well-thought-out meal plan, you can streamline your grocery shopping process, buy only the ingredients you need, and minimize food waste by using ingredients efficiently.

4. Reduces Stress and Decision-Making:
  - Meal planning reduces stress and decision fatigue associated with mealtime by eliminating the need to figure out what to eat on the spot.
  - Knowing what you'll be eating ahead of time allows you to prepare meals more efficiently, enjoy a sense of control over your food choices, and focus on other priorities throughout the day.

5. Encourages Variety and Creativity:
   - Meal planning encourages variety and creativity in your diet by exposing you to new recipes, flavors, and cooking techniques.
   - By experimenting with different ingredients and meal combinations, you can expand your culinary repertoire, discover new favorite dishes, and make mealtime more enjoyable and exciting.

6. Supports Portion Control:
   - Planning meals in advance can help individuals practice portion control and prevent overeating by pre-portioning meals and snacks according to their nutritional needs.
   - By being mindful of portion sizes and serving sizes when planning meals, you can prevent excessive calorie intake and maintain a healthy weight.

7. Enhances Food Security:
   - Meal planning can enhance food security by ensuring that individuals have access to nutritious meals and snacks throughout the week, even during busy or challenging times.
   - By having a plan in place, you can stock up on pantry staples, freezer-friendly ingredients, and shelf-stable foods to have on hand for quick and convenient meals.

8. Encourages Consistency and Routine:
   - Consistent meal planning fosters a sense of routine and structure around eating habits, which can promote healthier eating patterns and long-term dietary adherence.
   - By establishing regular meal times and planning meals in advance, you can create a sense of predictability and stability in your eating routine, making it easier to maintain healthy habits over time.

Building Nutrient-Dense Meals

Building nutrient-dense meals is essential for supporting overall health and well-being. Nutrient-dense meals provide a high concentration of essential vitamins, minerals, antioxidants, and other beneficial compounds while being relatively low in added sugars, unhealthy fats, and empty calories. Here's how to build nutrient-dense meals:

1. Base Meals Around Whole Foods:
- Start by selecting whole, minimally processed foods as the foundation of your meals. This includes fruits, vegetables, whole grains, lean proteins, legumes, nuts, and seeds.
- Choose a variety of colorful fruits and vegetables to provide a wide range of vitamins, minerals, and antioxidants.

2. Include Lean Proteins:
- Incorporate lean sources of protein into your meals, such as skinless poultry, fish, seafood, tofu, tempeh, beans, lentils, and low-fat dairy products.
- Protein is essential for muscle repair and growth, immune function, hormone production, and satiety.

3. Add Healthy Fats:
- Include sources of healthy fats in your meals, such as avocados, nuts, seeds, olive oil, fatty fish (e.g., salmon, mackerel), and flaxseeds.
- Healthy fats provide essential fatty acids (omega-3 and omega-6), promote heart health, and aid in the absorption of fat-soluble vitamins (A, D, E, K).

4. Choose Whole Grains:
- Opt for whole grains instead of refined grains to maximize nutrient intake and promote satiety. Examples include brown rice, quinoa, oats, barley, whole wheat pasta, and whole grain bread.
- Whole grains provide fiber, vitamins (e.g., B vitamins), minerals (e.g., magnesium, iron), and antioxidants.

5. Incorporate Colorful Fruits and Vegetables:
- Aim to fill half your plate with colorful fruits and vegetables at each meal. Choose a variety of colors to ensure you're getting a diverse range of nutrients.
- Colorful fruits and vegetables are rich in vitamins, minerals, fiber, and phytonutrients that support overall health and reduce the risk of chronic diseases.

6. Include Fiber-Rich Foods:

- Incorporate fiber-rich foods such as fruits, vegetables, whole grains, legumes, nuts, and seeds into your meals and snacks.
- Fiber supports digestive health, regulates blood sugar levels, promotes satiety, and reduces the risk of heart disease and certain cancers.

7. Limit Added Sugars and Processed Foods:

- Minimize the consumption of added sugars, refined grains, processed foods, and sugary beverages, which provide empty calories and lack essential nutrients.
- Instead, focus on whole, nutrient-dense foods that provide sustained energy and support overall health.

8. Prioritize Nutrient-Rich Snacks:

- Choose nutrient-rich snacks such as fresh fruit, raw vegetables with hummus, Greek yogurt with berries, nuts and seeds, or whole grain crackers with avocado and lean protein.
- Snacking on nutrient-dense foods helps to maintain energy levels, curb hunger between meals, and support overall nutrient intake.

9. Use Herbs and Spices for Flavor:

- Enhance the flavor of your meals with herbs, spices, and natural seasonings instead of relying on salt, sugar, or unhealthy condiments.
- Herbs and spices add depth and complexity to dishes while providing additional health benefits due to their antioxidant and anti-inflammatory properties.

10. Stay Hydrated:

- Don't forget the importance of hydration for overall health. Drink water throughout the day and limit consumption of sugary beverages and excessive caffeine.
- Hydration supports digestion, nutrient absorption, cognitive function, and overall well-being.

Cooking Methods for Healthy Eating

Cooking methods play a crucial role in determining the nutritional quality of meals. By choosing healthier cooking techniques, you can retain the nutrients in foods while minimizing the addition of unhealthy fats, sugars, and calories. Here are some cooking methods for healthy eating:

1. Grilling:
  - Grilling is a great way to cook lean proteins such as chicken, fish, tofu, and vegetables without adding extra fat.
  - Use a grill pan or an outdoor grill to cook foods over direct heat, resulting in a flavorful charred exterior while preserving the natural juices and nutrients inside.

2. Baking and Roasting:
  - Baking and roasting are gentle cooking methods that help retain the natural flavors and nutrients of foods.
  - Place foods such as chicken, fish, vegetables, and whole grains in the oven at a moderate temperature to cook them evenly and develop delicious caramelization.

3. Steaming:
  - Steaming is a gentle cooking method that preserves the color, texture, and nutritional value of vegetables, seafood, and grains.
  - Use a steamer basket or a steam oven to cook foods with minimal water, allowing them to retain their vitamins, minerals, and antioxidants.

4. Sauteing and Stir-Frying:
  - Sauteing and stir-frying involve cooking foods quickly in a small amount of healthy oil over high heat.
  - Use heart-healthy oils like olive oil, avocado oil, or coconut oil and incorporate plenty of colorful vegetables, lean proteins, and whole grains for a nutritious and flavorful meal.

5. Poaching:
  - Poaching involves gently simmering foods in liquid, such as water, broth, or wine, at a low temperature until they are cooked through.

- Poaching is an excellent method for cooking delicate proteins like fish, chicken, eggs, and fruits, preserving their moisture and tenderness.

6. Boiling and Simmering:
- Boiling and simmering are simple cooking methods that require submerging foods in water or broth and cooking them until tender.
- Use this method for cooking grains, legumes, pasta, and vegetables, being mindful not to overcook them to preserve their texture and nutrients.

7. Broiling:
- Broiling involves cooking foods under high heat in the oven, resulting in a crispy exterior and juicy interior.
- Use the broil setting to cook lean proteins like chicken or fish, as well as vegetables, until they are golden brown and caramelized.

8. Griddling:
- Griddling is a dry cooking method that involves cooking foods on a flat surface, such as a griddle pan or a grill pan, without the need for added fats.
- Use a griddle to cook vegetables, fruits, lean proteins, and whole grain bread for a quick and healthy meal option.

9. Slow Cooking:
- Slow cooking involves cooking foods over a long period at low temperatures, allowing flavors to develop and ingredients to tenderize.
- Use a slow cooker or crockpot to prepare soups, stews, chili, and braised meats, incorporating plenty of vegetables and lean proteins for a nutritious meal.

10. Microwaving:
- Microwaving is a convenient cooking method that can help preserve the nutrients in foods while reducing cooking time.
- Use the microwave to steam vegetables, cook grains, reheat leftovers, and prepare quick and healthy meals when time is limited.

Smart Snacking Choices

Smart snacking choices are an essential part of a healthy eating plan, providing nourishment between meals and helping to maintain energy levels throughout the day. Here are some guidelines for making smart snacking choices:

1. Choose Whole, Nutrient-Dense Foods:
- Opt for whole, minimally processed foods that are rich in nutrients and provide sustained energy. Examples include fruits, vegetables, nuts, seeds, whole grains, and lean proteins.
- Whole foods are typically higher in fiber, vitamins, minerals, and antioxidants compared to processed snack foods, which often contain added sugars, unhealthy fats, and empty calories.

2. Include a Balance of Macronutrients:
- Aim to include a balance of macronutrients in your snacks, including carbohydrates, proteins, and healthy fats, to promote satiety and provide sustained energy.
- Pairing carbohydrate-rich foods like fruits or whole grains with protein-rich options like nuts or Greek yogurt can help stabilize blood sugar levels and prevent energy crashes.

3. Practice Portion Control:
- Be mindful of portion sizes when snacking to avoid overeating and consuming excess calories. Use small bowls or containers to portion out snacks and avoid eating directly from the package.
- Aim for a balance between satisfying your hunger and preventing excessive calorie intake, especially if weight management is a concern.

4. Plan Ahead and Prepare Snacks:
- Plan ahead by preparing healthy snacks in advance and keeping them readily available for when hunger strikes. This can help prevent impulsive food choices and reduce the temptation to reach for less nutritious options.
- Consider batch-prepping snacks like chopped fruits and vegetables, homemade trail mix, Greek yogurt parfaits, or hard-boiled eggs to have on hand throughout the week.

5. Focus on Whole Fruits and Vegetables:

- Whole fruits and vegetables make convenient and nutritious snack choices, providing essential vitamins, minerals, fiber, and hydration.
- Enjoy fresh fruits and vegetables on their own or pair them with protein or healthy fats for a balanced snack. Examples include apple slices with almond butter, carrot sticks with hummus, or cucumber slices with cottage cheese.

6. Incorporate Protein-Rich Options:
- Including protein-rich foods in your snacks can help promote satiety and support muscle repair and growth. Choose lean protein sources such as Greek yogurt, cottage cheese, hard-boiled eggs, edamame, or turkey slices.
- Protein-rich snacks can help keep you feeling full and satisfied between meals, reducing the likelihood of overeating later in the day.

7. Opt for Healthy Fats:
- Healthy fats provide essential fatty acids and help increase the satisfaction and palatability of snacks. Choose options like nuts, seeds, avocado, olives, or nut butter to add healthy fats to your snacks.
- Incorporating small amounts of healthy fats into your snacks can help keep you feeling satisfied and prevent cravings for less nutritious foods.

8. Read Labels and Avoid Added Sugars and Unhealthy Fats:
- When choosing packaged snacks, read the ingredient labels and nutrition facts to avoid options that are high in added sugars, unhealthy fats, and artificial additives.
- Look for snacks with minimal ingredients, whole food sources, and no added sugars or artificial sweeteners to support your health goals and provide sustained energy.

9. Stay Hydrated:
- Don't forget the importance of hydration when snacking. Opt for water, herbal tea, or infused water as your beverage of choice to stay hydrated and support overall well-being.
- Drinking water alongside snacks can help enhance satiety and prevent thirst from being mistaken for hunger.

10. Listen to Your Body:

- Pay attention to your hunger and fullness cues when snacking, and eat mindfully to avoid mindless eating.
- Choose snacks that satisfy your hunger and provide nourishment, rather than eating out of boredom, stress, or habit.

Preparing Balanced Meals on a Budget

Preparing balanced meals on a budget is not only feasible but also essential for maintaining a healthy diet without breaking the bank. Here are some strategies for achieving this:

1. Plan Meals and Create a Shopping List:
- Plan your meals for the week ahead of time to avoid impulse purchases and wastage. Take inventory of what you already have in your pantry and fridge.
- Create a shopping list based on your meal plan and stick to it while grocery shopping to avoid buying unnecessary items.

2. Choose Inexpensive Protein Sources:
- Opt for budget-friendly protein sources such as canned beans, lentils, eggs, canned tuna, tofu, and frozen chicken breasts or thighs.
- These options provide essential nutrients like protein, vitamins, and minerals at a lower cost compared to more expensive cuts of meat or seafood.

3. Buy Whole Foods in Bulk:
- Purchase whole foods like grains (rice, oats, quinoa), legumes (beans, lentils), and pasta in bulk quantities. Buying in bulk often results in lower per-unit costs.
- Store bulk items in airtight containers to maintain freshness and prevent spoilage.

4. Embrace Frozen and Canned Produce:
- Frozen and canned fruits and vegetables are budget-friendly options that are just as nutritious as fresh produce and have a longer shelf life.
- Stock up on frozen vegetables, berries, and canned tomatoes, beans, and corn to incorporate into meals like soups, stir-fries, and smoothies.

5. Cook in Batches and Freeze Portions:

- Cook large batches of meals like soups, stews, casseroles, and grains and freeze individual portions for later use.
- This not only saves time but also prevents food waste by ensuring leftovers are used before they spoil.

6. Focus on Seasonal and Sale Items:

- Purchase seasonal fruits and vegetables when they are abundant and therefore cheaper. Seasonal produce tends to be fresher and more flavorful.
- Take advantage of sales and discounts on staple items like grains, canned goods, and frozen foods to save money.

7. Use Affordable Flavor Boosters:

- Enhance the flavor of budget-friendly meals with inexpensive ingredients like herbs, spices, garlic, onions, vinegar, and citrus juice.
- These flavor boosters can transform simple dishes into delicious and satisfying meals without the need for expensive sauces or seasonings.

8. Limit Processed and Convenience Foods:

- Minimize purchases of processed and convenience foods, which are often more expensive and less nutritious than homemade options.
- Cooking from scratch allows you to control the ingredients and portion sizes, resulting in healthier and more budget-friendly meals.

9. Repurpose Leftovers:

- Get creative with leftovers by repurposing them into new meals. For example, leftover roasted vegetables can be added to salads, soups, or omelets, while cooked grains can be turned into grain bowls or stir-fries.
- This reduces food waste and saves money by making the most out of what you already have on hand.

10. Compare Prices and Shop Smart:

- Compare prices between different grocery stores and consider shopping at discount supermarkets or using coupons and loyalty programs to save money.

- Look for store-brand or generic versions of products, which are often cheaper than name-brand items without sacrificing quality.

Chapter 8
Understanding Food Labels

Reading and Interpreting Nutrition Labels

Reading and interpreting nutrition labels is essential for making informed food choices and selecting products that align with your dietary goals and preferences. Here's a step-by-step guide to reading and understanding nutrition labels:

1. Start with the Serving Size:
- The serving size indicates the amount of food or beverage typically consumed at one time and is listed at the top of the nutrition label.
- Pay attention to the serving size, as all the nutrient information on the label is based on this amount.

2. Check the Number of Servings per Container:
- Next to the serving size, you'll find the number of servings per container or package.
- Multiply the number of servings by the amount you typically consume to determine the total nutrient intake if you eat the entire package.

3. Review the Calories:
- The calorie count per serving provides information about the energy content of the food.
- Consider your individual calorie needs and the serving size to determine how many calories you'll consume from the product.

4. Examine Macronutrients:
- Look at the amounts of macronutrients (carbohydrates, proteins, and fats) listed on the label.
- Pay attention to the grams of each macronutrient per serving and consider your dietary goals and preferences. For example, choose products with higher protein and fiber content for increased satiety.

5. Assess % Daily Value (%DV):
- %DV indicates how much a serving of the food contributes to your daily nutrient intake based on a 2,000-calorie diet.
- Aim to choose foods with higher %DV of nutrients like fiber, vitamins, and minerals (e.g., calcium, iron) and lower %DV of nutrients like saturated fat, sodium, and added sugars.

6. Limit Saturated Fat, Trans Fat, Sodium, and Added Sugars:
   - Pay attention to the amounts of saturated fat, trans fat, sodium, and added sugars listed on the label.
   - Limit intake of these nutrients, as excessive consumption may increase the risk of chronic diseases such as heart disease, hypertension, and obesity.

7. Check Ingredient List:
   - Ingredients are listed in descending order by weight, with the main ingredient listed first.
   - Choose products with fewer ingredients and recognize and avoid additives, preservatives, and artificial sweeteners if desired.

8. Consider Additional Nutrients:
   - Some nutrition labels may include additional nutrients like vitamins, minerals, fiber, or other beneficial compounds.
   - Look for products that provide essential nutrients and contribute to a balanced diet.

9. Be Aware of Health Claims:
   - Pay attention to health claims on the packaging, such as "low-fat," "high-fiber," or "reduced sodium."
   - Be cautious and evaluate the overall nutrient content of the product, as some claims may be misleading or only apply to specific nutrients.

10. Compare Similar Products:
   - When choosing between similar products, compare the nutrient content, serving sizes, and ingredient lists to make the best choice for your nutritional needs and preferences.

Identifying Hidden Sugars and Additives

Identifying hidden sugars and additives on food labels is crucial for making informed choices about your dietary intake and avoiding excessive consumption of these ingredients, which can have negative effects on health. Here's how to identify hidden sugars and additives on food labels:

1. Look for Various Names for Sugar:

- Sugar can be listed under various names on food labels, including sucrose, glucose, fructose, high-fructose corn syrup (HFCS), corn syrup, maltose, dextrose, honey, molasses, and cane sugar.
- Check the ingredient list for these terms to identify added sugars in products.

2. Check for Artificial Sweeteners:

- Artificial sweeteners are sugar substitutes that provide sweetness without the calories of sugar. Look for names such as aspartame, saccharin, sucralose, acesulfame potassium (Ace-K), and neotame in the ingredient list.
- While artificial sweeteners are low in calories, some studies suggest they may have negative health effects when consumed in excess.

3. Be Mindful of Hidden Sugars in "Health" Foods:

- Even products marketed as "healthy" or "natural" may contain hidden sugars. Check the nutrition label and ingredient list for added sugars in products like yogurt, granola bars, cereals, salad dressings, and flavored beverages.
- Choose unsweetened or minimally processed versions of these foods whenever possible.

4. Watch Out for Hidden Sources of Added Sugars:

- Some products may contain added sugars in unexpected forms, such as sauces, condiments, flavored yogurts, and canned or packaged foods.
- Check the ingredient list for sources of added sugars and choose products with little to no added sugars or opt for homemade versions with healthier sweeteners like fruit, honey, or maple syrup.

5. Avoid Artificial Additives:

- Scan the ingredient list for artificial additives, preservatives, colorings, and flavorings, which may have adverse effects on health.
- Look for terms like artificial flavors, artificial colors (e.g., FD&C Yellow No. 5), artificial preservatives (e.g., BHA, BHT), and

monosodium glutamate (MSG), and choose products without these additives whenever possible.

6. Be Wary of Highly Processed Foods:
   - Highly processed foods often contain hidden sugars, additives, and other undesirable ingredients. These foods may contribute to weight gain, inflammation, and chronic diseases when consumed in excess.
   - Choose whole, minimally processed foods whenever possible and limit intake of processed snacks, desserts, and convenience foods.

7. Check for "Low-Fat" or "Fat-Free" Claims:
   - Products labeled as "low-fat" or "fat-free" may contain added sugars and other additives to enhance flavor and texture.
   - Pay attention to the ingredient list and nutrition label to ensure that these products don't contain excessive amounts of added sugars or unhealthy additives.

8. Be Skeptical of Marketing Claims:
   - Be skeptical of marketing claims like "all-natural," "organic," or "healthy," as these terms do not necessarily indicate the absence of hidden sugars or additives.
   - Always check the ingredient list and nutrition label to verify the nutritional content of the product.

9. Read Food Labels Carefully:
   - Take the time to read food labels carefully and familiarize yourself with common names for sugars and additives.
   - Look for products with simple ingredient lists containing recognizable, whole food ingredients and minimal added sugars and artificial additives.

10. Make Informed Choices:
   - Use the information on food labels to make informed choices about your dietary intake and prioritize whole, nutrient-dense foods over highly processed products.
   - By identifying hidden sugars and additives on food labels, you can make healthier choices that support your overall health and well-being.

Making Informed Decisions at the Grocery Store

Making informed decisions at the grocery store involves understanding food labels, comparing products, and choosing foods that align with your nutritional goals and preferences. Here are some tips for making informed decisions while grocery shopping:

1. Plan Ahead:
  - Before heading to the store, create a shopping list based on your meal plan for the week. This will help you stay focused and avoid impulse purchases.

2. Read Food Labels:
  - Take the time to read and understand food labels, paying attention to serving sizes, calorie counts, macronutrient content, and ingredient lists.
  - Look for products with simple ingredient lists containing whole, minimally processed ingredients and avoid items with long lists of artificial additives, preservatives, and added sugars.

3. Compare Products:
  - Compare similar products to find the healthiest options. Look at the nutrition labels and ingredient lists to assess differences in nutrient content and quality.
  - Consider factors such as price, nutritional value, portion sizes, and packaging when comparing products.

4. Choose Whole Foods:
  - Focus on purchasing whole foods like fruits, vegetables, whole grains, lean proteins, and healthy fats. These foods are generally more nutritious and less processed than packaged and processed foods.
  - Prioritize fresh, seasonal produce, and opt for whole grains, lean meats, and minimally processed dairy products.

5. Shop the Perimeter:
  - In many grocery stores, the perimeter is where you'll find fresh produce, meats, dairy, and other whole foods. Spend most of your time shopping in these areas to prioritize nutritious options.

- Limit time spent in the center aisles, where processed and packaged foods are often located.

6. Be Skeptical of Marketing Claims:

- Be wary of marketing claims like "all-natural," "organic," or "low-fat," as these terms don't always indicate a healthier option.
- Look beyond front-of-package claims and read food labels carefully to verify the nutritional content of products.

7. Pay Attention to Portions:

- Consider portion sizes when selecting products, especially items that are easy to overeat, such as snacks and pre-packaged meals.
- Opt for single-serving portions or portion out larger packages into smaller containers to avoid overconsumption.

8. Be Flexible:

- Be open to trying new foods and experimenting with different recipes and ingredients. Variety is key to a balanced diet, so don't be afraid to explore new flavors and cuisines.
- Incorporate a variety of fruits, vegetables, whole grains, proteins, and healthy fats into your shopping cart to ensure you're getting a diverse range of nutrients.

9. Shop with a Budget in Mind:

- Set a budget for your grocery shopping trip and stick to it as much as possible. Look for sales, discounts, and bulk options to stretch your food dollars.
- Consider purchasing store-brand or generic versions of products, which are often more affordable than name-brand options without sacrificing quality.

10. Plan for Healthy Snacks:

- Stock up on nutritious snacks like fruits, vegetables, nuts, seeds, yogurt, and whole grain crackers to have on hand for when hunger strikes.
- Avoid impulse purchases of unhealthy snacks by planning ahead and having healthy options readily available.

The Importance of Portion Awareness

Portion awareness is crucial for maintaining a healthy diet and managing calorie intake. Understanding portion sizes allows you to control your food intake, prevent overeating, and make healthier choices. Here's why portion awareness is important when interpreting food labels and making dietary decisions:

1. Calorie Control:
  - Being aware of portion sizes helps you manage your calorie intake more effectively. Even nutritious foods can contribute to weight gain if consumed in excessive portions.
  - By understanding appropriate serving sizes, you can better gauge how much food you're consuming and avoid consuming more calories than your body needs.

2. Prevents Overeating:
  - Overeating, even on healthy foods, can lead to weight gain and other health issues over time. Large portion sizes can trick your brain into consuming more calories than necessary.
  - Portion awareness helps you recognize when you've had enough to eat and prevents mindless eating or eating beyond your hunger cues.

3. Supports Weight Management:
  - Maintaining a healthy weight is essential for overall health and well-being. Portion awareness can aid in weight management by ensuring you consume appropriate amounts of food to meet your energy needs.
  - By moderating portion sizes, you can create a calorie deficit or balance that supports weight loss, maintenance, or gain, depending on your goals.

4. Improves Nutrient Balance:
  - Consuming appropriate portion sizes allows for a more balanced intake of nutrients. Overeating one nutrient while neglecting others can lead to nutritional imbalances and deficiencies.
  - Portion awareness helps you distribute your food intake more evenly across macronutrients (carbohydrates, proteins, and fats) and micronutrients (vitamins and minerals).

5. Enhances Mindful Eating:
   - Portion awareness promotes mindful eating, which involves paying attention to hunger and fullness cues, as well as the sensory experience of eating.
   - By being mindful of portion sizes, you can savor your food, enjoy the flavors and textures, and cultivate a healthier relationship with food.

6. Reduces Food Waste:
   - Understanding portion sizes can help minimize food waste by preventing excess food from being prepared or consumed.
   - By portioning out appropriate amounts of food, you can avoid cooking or purchasing more than you need and reduce the likelihood of leftovers being thrown away.

7. Supports Sustainable Eating Habits:
   - Practicing portion awareness promotes sustainable eating habits that are realistic and maintainable in the long term.
   - By learning to listen to your body's hunger and fullness signals and eating appropriate portion sizes, you can develop a healthier relationship with food and avoid restrictive or unsustainable dieting practices.

8. Encourages Balanced Meals:
   - Portion awareness encourages the consumption of balanced meals that include a variety of nutrient-rich foods from all food groups.
   - By portioning out appropriate amounts of fruits, vegetables, whole grains, lean proteins, and healthy fats, you can create meals that provide essential nutrients and support overall health.

9. Empowers Informed Food Choices:
   - Being aware of portion sizes empowers you to make informed food choices based on your individual nutritional needs and goals.
   - When interpreting food labels, portion awareness helps you assess serving sizes and determine whether a product fits into your dietary plan.

10. Promotes Long-Term Health:

- Developing portion awareness is a valuable skill that supports long-term health and wellness. It allows you to enjoy a balanced diet, maintain a healthy weight, and reduce the risk of chronic diseases associated with overeating and poor dietary habits.

Using Food Labels to Meet Dietary Goals

Using food labels to meet dietary goals involves understanding how to interpret the information provided and making informed choices that align with your nutritional needs and preferences. Here's how to use food labels effectively to support your dietary goals:

1. Identify Key Nutrients:
- Determine which nutrients are important for your dietary goals, whether it's limiting sodium, sugar, or saturated fat, increasing fiber or protein intake, or monitoring calorie content.
- Use food labels to identify the amounts of these nutrients in the products you're considering.

2. Pay Attention to Serving Sizes:
- Check the serving size listed on the food label to ensure it matches the portion you plan to consume. Serving sizes can vary significantly between products and may not always reflect typical portion sizes.
- Adjust the nutrient values accordingly based on your intended portion size.

3. Compare Products:
- Compare similar products to find options that best meet your dietary goals. Look at the nutrition facts panel and ingredient lists to assess differences in nutrient content and quality.
- Consider factors such as calorie content, macronutrient composition, fiber content, and the presence of additives or preservatives.

4. Monitor Calorie Intake:
- Use food labels to track your calorie intake and ensure it aligns with your calorie goals for weight maintenance, loss, or gain.

- Pay attention to the calorie count per serving and adjust portion sizes accordingly to stay within your calorie targets.

5. Limit Unhealthy Nutrients:
- Be mindful of nutrients to limit, such as saturated fat, trans fat, cholesterol, sodium, and added sugars. Use food labels to identify products that are lower in these nutrients or contain healthier alternatives.
- Look for products labeled as "low-fat," "low-sodium," or "no added sugars" to help guide your choices.

6. Choose Nutrient-Dense Foods:
- Opt for nutrient-dense foods that provide essential vitamins, minerals, and other beneficial nutrients without excessive calories, sugars, or unhealthy fats.
- Look for foods that are rich in nutrients like fiber, vitamins, and minerals and low in added sugars, sodium, and unhealthy fats.

7. Prioritize Whole Foods:
- Choose whole, minimally processed foods whenever possible, as they tend to be higher in nutrients and lower in unhealthy additives.
- Look for products with short ingredient lists containing recognizable, whole food ingredients and minimal added sugars, artificial additives, or preservatives.

8. Read Ingredient Lists:
- Check the ingredient list to understand what's in the product and prioritize foods with simple, wholesome ingredients.
- Be cautious of products with long lists of artificial additives, preservatives, or unfamiliar ingredients, as they may not align with your dietary goals.

9. Consider Dietary Restrictions:
- If you have dietary restrictions or special dietary needs (e.g., gluten-free, dairy-free, vegetarian, vegan), use food labels to identify products that meet your requirements.
- Look for products labeled as suitable for your dietary preferences or carefully review ingredient lists for potential allergens or prohibited ingredients.

10. Be Mindful of Marketing Claims:
   - Be critical of marketing claims on food packaging and use food labels as a tool to verify the nutritional content of products.
   - Look beyond front-of-package claims and read the nutrition facts panel and ingredient list to make informed decisions about the products you choose to purchase and consume.

Chapter 9
Hydration and Its Impact on Health

The Importance of Staying Hydrated

The importance of staying hydrated cannot be overstated, as adequate hydration is essential for overall health and well-being. Here are several reasons why staying hydrated is crucial:

1. Maintains Fluid Balance:
   - Water makes up a significant portion of your body, including cells, tissues, and organs. Staying hydrated helps maintain fluid balance, which is essential for various bodily functions, including digestion, circulation, temperature regulation, and nutrient transport.

2. Supports Proper Digestion:
   - Drinking enough water is crucial for proper digestion and nutrient absorption. Water helps dissolve and transport nutrients, aids in the breakdown of food particles, and supports the movement of food through the digestive tract.

3. Regulates Body Temperature:
   - Sweating is the body's natural mechanism for regulating temperature and preventing overheating during physical activity or exposure to heat. Staying hydrated helps replenish lost fluids through sweating and maintains optimal body temperature.

4. Supports Kidney Function:
   - Adequate hydration is vital for proper kidney function and urinary health. Water helps flush waste products and toxins from the body through urine, preventing the buildup of harmful substances in the kidneys and urinary tract.

5. Promotes Cardiovascular Health:
   - Proper hydration supports cardiovascular health by maintaining adequate blood volume and circulation. Dehydration can lead to reduced blood volume, increased heart rate, and decreased blood pressure, putting added strain on the heart and increasing the risk of cardiovascular issues.

6. Enhances Physical Performance:

- Staying hydrated is crucial for optimal physical performance and exercise endurance. Dehydration can lead to fatigue, muscle cramps, and reduced exercise capacity, impairing performance and recovery.
- Drinking enough water before, during, and after physical activity helps maintain hydration levels and supports peak performance.

7. Improves Cognitive Function:
- Hydration plays a significant role in cognitive function and mental clarity. Dehydration can impair concentration, memory, and mood, leading to decreased alertness and cognitive performance.
- Drinking water regularly throughout the day helps keep the brain hydrated and supports optimal cognitive function and productivity.

8. Boosts Energy Levels:
- Adequate hydration is essential for maintaining energy levels and combating fatigue. Dehydration can lead to feelings of tiredness, lethargy, and reduced mental and physical stamina.
- Drinking water helps replenish lost fluids, supports nutrient delivery to cells, and provides a natural energy boost to keep you feeling alert and energized.

9. Supports Skin Health:
- Staying hydrated promotes healthy skin by maintaining moisture levels, improving elasticity, and reducing the risk of dryness, irritation, and premature aging.
- Dehydration can lead to dull, dry skin, exacerbate skin conditions like acne and eczema, and contribute to the formation of wrinkles and fine lines.

10. Aids in Weight Management:
- Drinking water can support weight management goals by promoting feelings of fullness and reducing calorie intake. Staying hydrated can help prevent overeating and snacking, support healthy metabolism, and enhance the body's ability to burn fat.

Water vs. Sugary Beverages

Comparing water to sugary beverages highlights significant differences in their impact on health. Here's a breakdown of the key differences:

1. Hydration:
   - Water: Water is the optimal choice for hydration as it is calorie-free and readily absorbed by the body. It effectively replenishes fluids lost through sweat, urine, and respiration, supporting overall hydration and bodily functions.
   - Sugary Beverages: Sugary beverages like soda, fruit juice, energy drinks, and sweetened teas often contain added sugars and calories, which provide energy but do not contribute to hydration. In fact, the high sugar content in these beverages can lead to increased thirst and may even contribute to dehydration when consumed in excess.

2. Caloric Content:
   - Water: Water contains zero calories, making it an ideal choice for those looking to manage their weight or reduce calorie intake. It satisfies thirst without adding extra calories to the diet.
   - Sugary Beverages: Sugary beverages are high in calories due to added sugars, which contribute to weight gain and can increase the risk of obesity, diabetes, and other chronic diseases when consumed in excess. Regular consumption of sugary beverages can contribute to an imbalance in calorie intake and expenditure, leading to weight gain over time.

3. Nutrient Content:
   - Water: Water is devoid of nutrients, providing only hydration without any additional vitamins, minerals, or macronutrients. While it is essential for overall health, water does not contribute to nutrient intake.
   - Sugary Beverages: Sugary beverages typically lack essential nutrients and provide empty calories derived from added sugars. They offer little nutritional value beyond energy and can displace more nutrient-dense beverages like water, milk, or unsweetened teas.

4. Blood Sugar Impact:
   - Water: Water has no effect on blood sugar levels as it contains no carbohydrates or sugars. It is suitable for individuals with diabetes or those looking to manage blood sugar levels.

- Sugary Beverages: Sugary beverages can cause rapid spikes in blood sugar levels due to their high sugar content. This can lead to fluctuations in energy levels, mood swings, and increased risk of insulin resistance and type 2 diabetes, particularly with frequent consumption.

5. Dental Health:
- Water: Water is beneficial for dental health as it helps rinse away food particles, bacteria, and acids that can contribute to tooth decay and gum disease. Drinking water throughout the day can help maintain oral hygiene and reduce the risk of cavities.
- Sugary Beverages: Sugary beverages are a significant contributor to tooth decay and dental erosion due to their high sugar and acid content. Regular consumption can lead to cavities, enamel erosion, and other oral health issues, especially when combined with poor dental hygiene practices.

6. Satiety and Hunger Regulation:
- Water: Drinking water can promote feelings of fullness and satiety, helping to curb appetite and prevent overeating. It is an excellent choice for staying hydrated between meals and reducing snacking.
- Sugary Beverages: Sugary beverages provide little satiety despite their high calorie content. The rapid absorption of liquid calories may not trigger the same feelings of fullness as solid foods, leading to increased calorie consumption and potential weight gain.

Signs of Dehydration and Overhydration

Recognizing signs of dehydration and overhydration is crucial for maintaining optimal hydration levels and overall health. Here's a breakdown of the signs and symptoms associated with each condition:

Signs of Dehydration:

1. Thirst: Feeling thirsty is one of the earliest signs of dehydration. It's your body's way of signaling that it needs more fluids.
2. Dark Urine: Dark yellow or amber-colored urine is a sign of concentrated urine, indicating dehydration. Inadequate fluid intake leads to reduced urine output and darker urine.

3. Dry Mouth and Lips: Dehydration can cause dryness in the mouth and lips due to reduced saliva production.

4. Fatigue and Weakness: Dehydration can lead to feelings of tiredness, weakness, and lethargy as the body's energy levels decrease.

5. Headache: Dehydration can trigger headaches and migraines due to changes in blood volume and electrolyte balance.

6. Dizziness or Lightheadedness: Dehydration can cause dizziness, lightheadedness, and fainting episodes due to reduced blood flow to the brain.

7. Reduced Urination: Infrequent urination or a significant decrease in urine output is a sign of dehydration.

8. Dry Skin: Dehydration can lead to dry, flaky skin and a lack of elasticity due to reduced moisture levels.

9. Muscle Cramps: Dehydration can cause muscle cramps, spasms, or weakness due to imbalances in electrolytes like sodium, potassium, and magnesium.

10. Rapid Heart Rate: Dehydration can lead to an increased heart rate or heart palpitations as the body tries to compensate for reduced blood volume.

Signs of Overhydration:

1. Excessive Urination: Overhydration can lead to frequent urination and an increased volume of dilute urine, often clear or pale yellow in color.

2. Swelling or Edema: Overhydration can cause swelling or edema, particularly in the hands, feet, ankles, or abdomen, due to fluid retention.

3. Nausea and Vomiting: Overhydration may cause nausea, vomiting, or gastrointestinal discomfort as the body tries to expel excess fluids.

4. Headache: Similar to dehydration, overhydration can also trigger headaches or migraines due to shifts in fluid and electrolyte balance.

5. Confusion or Disorientation: Overhydration can lead to confusion, disorientation, or changes in mental status due to imbalances in electrolytes like sodium.

6. Fatigue and Weakness: Overhydration may cause feelings of fatigue, weakness, or lethargy as electrolyte imbalances affect energy levels.

7. Muscle Cramps: In severe cases, overhydration can lead to muscle cramps, spasms, or weakness due to electrolyte disturbances.

8. Hyponatremia: Overhydration can result in low blood sodium levels (hyponatremia), which can cause symptoms like nausea, headache, confusion, seizures, or coma if left untreated.
9. Bloating or Fullness: Overhydration may cause feelings of bloating, fullness, or discomfort in the stomach due to excess fluid in the digestive tract.
10. Weight Gain: Over time, chronic overhydration may lead to weight gain due to fluid retention and imbalances in fluid distribution within the body.

It's essential to listen to your body and pay attention to these signs and symptoms to maintain proper hydration levels. If you experience symptoms of dehydration or overhydration, it's essential to adjust your fluid intake accordingly and seek medical attention if symptoms persist or worsen.

Calculating Daily Water Needs

Calculating your daily water needs involves considering various factors such as age, gender, body weight, activity level, climate, and overall health. While individual water needs can vary significantly, there are general guidelines to help you estimate how much water you should be drinking each day. Here's how to calculate your daily water needs:

1. Use the Adequate Intake (AI) Recommendations:
   - The AI for total water intake includes water from beverages and foods and is as follows:
      - Adult Men: About 3.7 liters (125 ounces) per day
      - Adult Women: About 2.7 liters (91 ounces) per day

2. Adjust for Individual Factors:
   - Consider factors that may increase your water needs, such as:
   - Body Weight: Larger individuals generally require more water to stay hydrated.
   - Physical Activity: Sweating during exercise increases fluid loss and necessitates higher water intake.
   - Climate: Hot and humid weather or high altitudes can increase fluid loss through sweat and respiration.

- Pregnancy or Breastfeeding: Pregnant or breastfeeding individuals require additional water to support maternal and fetal hydration needs.

3. Calculate Based on Body Weight:

- A commonly used method to estimate water needs is to consume about 30-35 milliliters (1-1.2 ounces) of water per kilogram of body weight.
- For example, a person weighing 70 kilograms (154 pounds) would require approximately 2.1-2.45 liters (70-83 ounces) of water per day.

4. Monitor Hydration Status:

- Pay attention to signs of dehydration, such as thirst, dark urine, dry mouth, fatigue, and dizziness. Adjust your water intake accordingly based on your hydration status and activity level.
- Consider factors like sweating, urination frequency, and overall fluid balance to gauge your hydration needs throughout the day.

5. Adjust for Fluid Losses:

- Account for fluid losses due to factors like sweating, urination, and respiration. If you engage in strenuous physical activity or spend time in hot or humid environments, you may need to increase your water intake to compensate for increased fluid loss.

6. Consider Dietary Sources of Water:

- Remember that water intake includes not only plain water but also fluids from other beverages (e.g., tea, coffee, milk, juice) and water-rich foods (e.g., fruits, vegetables, soups).
- Incorporate hydrating foods and beverages into your diet to help meet your daily water needs.

7. Listen to Your Body:

- Pay attention to your body's thirst signals and drink water whenever you feel thirsty. Thirst is a reliable indicator of fluid needs and should not be ignored.
- Additionally, aim to maintain pale or light-colored urine throughout the day as a sign of adequate hydration.

8. Be Flexible:

- Individual water needs can vary based on factors like age, health status, and environmental conditions. Adjust your water intake as needed to meet your unique hydration needs and preferences.

Enhancing Hydration Through Healthy Beverages

Enhancing hydration through healthy beverages involves choosing fluids that not only quench your thirst but also provide essential nutrients and support overall health. Here are several options for healthy beverages that can help you stay hydrated:

1. Water:
- Water is the best choice for staying hydrated, as it contains zero calories and is readily absorbed by the body. Drink plain water throughout the day to maintain hydration levels and support bodily functions.

2. Herbal Tea:
- Herbal teas are caffeine-free and can be enjoyed hot or cold. Choose herbal teas like chamomile, peppermint, or ginger for a hydrating and soothing beverage option.
- Avoid adding sugar or sweeteners to herbal teas to keep them calorie-free and maintain their hydrating properties.

3. Infused Water:
- Infuse water with fresh fruits, vegetables, or herbs to add flavor and encourage hydration. Try combinations like cucumber and mint, lemon and basil, or berries and citrus for a refreshing twist.
- Infused water provides natural flavor without added sugars or calories, making it a hydrating and flavorful beverage option.

4. Coconut Water:
- Coconut water is a natural source of electrolytes like potassium and magnesium, making it an excellent choice for hydration, particularly after exercise or in hot weather.
- Look for unsweetened coconut water to avoid added sugars and unnecessary calories.

5. Vegetable Juice:

- Vegetable juices like tomato, cucumber, or carrot juice can be hydrating and nutrient-rich options. Vegetable juices provide vitamins, minerals, and antioxidants while also contributing to hydration.
- Choose low-sodium vegetable juices and limit the addition of high-sodium ingredients like salt or vegetable broth to maintain a healthy balance.

6. Fruit Smoothies:

- Fruit smoothies made with water, yogurt, or milk and blended with fresh or frozen fruits can be hydrating and nutritious. Smoothies provide hydration along with vitamins, minerals, fiber, and antioxidants from fruits and other ingredients.
- Use whole fruits or vegetables in smoothies rather than fruit juices or sweetened concentrates to maximize nutritional value and minimize added sugars.

7. Low-Fat Milk or Plant-Based Milk Alternatives:

- Low-fat milk and plant-based milk alternatives like almond, soy, or oat milk are hydrating options that provide calcium, vitamin D, and other essential nutrients.
- Choose unsweetened varieties of plant-based milk and limit added sugars to keep them a healthy beverage choice.

8. Electrolyte Drinks (in Moderation):

- Electrolyte drinks like sports drinks or electrolyte-enhanced water can help replenish electrolytes lost through sweating during intense physical activity or in hot weather.
- However, these beverages may contain added sugars and calories, so consume them in moderation and reserve them for situations where electrolyte replacement is necessary.

9. Green Tea:

- Green tea is a hydrating beverage that contains antioxidants called catechins, which may have various health benefits. Enjoy green tea hot or cold for a refreshing and hydrating drink option.
- Opt for unsweetened green tea to avoid added sugars and maximize its health-promoting properties.

10. Sparkling Water:
   - Sparkling water or seltzer water can be a refreshing and hydrating alternative to plain water. Choose unsweetened sparkling water and add a splash of lemon or lime juice for extra flavor without added sugars.
   - Be cautious of flavored sparkling water varieties that may contain added sugars or artificial sweeteners. Opt for natural flavors or plain sparkling water whenever possible.

Chapter 10
Special Considerations: Nutrition Across the Lifespan

Nutrition for Infants and Toddlers

Nutrition for infants and toddlers is critical for healthy growth and development during this crucial stage of life. Here are some essential considerations for ensuring proper nutrition for infants and toddlers:

1. Breastfeeding or Formula Feeding:
   - Breastfeeding is recommended as the best source of nutrition for infants during the first six months of life. Breast milk provides essential nutrients, antibodies, and enzymes that support immune function and healthy growth.
   - If breastfeeding is not possible or insufficient, infant formula is a suitable alternative. Choose commercially prepared infant formulas that meet the nutritional needs of infants and are safe for consumption.

2. Introduction of Solid Foods:
   - The American Academy of Pediatrics recommends introducing solid foods around six months of age, in addition to breast milk or formula. Start with single-ingredient, iron-fortified infant cereals, pureed fruits, vegetables, and meats.
   - Gradually introduce a variety of textures and flavors to expand your child's palate and provide a balanced diet.

3. Nutrient-Rich Foods:
   - Offer a variety of nutrient-rich foods to support healthy growth and development. Include foods rich in iron, zinc, calcium, vitamin D, vitamin C, and healthy fats.
   - Offer a variety of fruits, vegetables, whole grains, lean proteins, dairy or dairy alternatives, and healthy fats in age-appropriate portions.

4. Portion Sizes and Feeding Schedule:
   - Pay attention to portion sizes and feeding schedules appropriate for your child's age and developmental stage. Offer small, frequent meals and snacks throughout the day to meet your child's energy and nutrient needs.
   - Let your child's hunger and fullness cues guide feeding times and portion sizes, and avoid pressuring or forcing them to eat.

5. Food Safety:
   - Practice proper food safety and hygiene when preparing, handling, and storing food for infants and toddlers. Wash hands thoroughly before handling food, and ensure utensils and feeding equipment are clean and sanitized.
   - Avoid giving infants and toddlers foods that pose a choking hazard, such as whole grapes, nuts, popcorn, hard candies, and chunks of raw vegetables.

6. Limit Added Sugars and Salt:
   - Minimize the intake of added sugars and salt in your child's diet. Offer foods with natural sweetness from fruits and limit the consumption of sugary snacks, desserts, and sweetened beverages.
   - Avoid adding salt or salty seasonings to your child's food and opt for natural herbs and spices to flavor meals instead.

7. Encourage Self-Feeding and Independence:
   - Encourage self-feeding and independence during meals and snacks as your child grows. Offer age-appropriate utensils and serving dishes and allow your child to explore and experiment with different foods and textures.
   - Supervise meal times and offer guidance and support as needed, but allow your child to develop self-feeding skills and autonomy.

8. Seek Professional Guidance:
   - Consult with a pediatrician or registered dietitian if you have questions or concerns about your child's nutrition, growth, or feeding habits. They can provide personalized recommendations and support to ensure your child receives adequate nutrition for optimal growth and development.

Childhood Nutrition: Building Healthy Habits

Childhood nutrition plays a crucial role in shaping long-term health and well-being. By building healthy eating habits early in life, children can develop a strong foundation for optimal growth, development, and overall health. Here are some essential considerations for promoting healthy eating habits in children:

1. Role Modeling:
   - Set a positive example by modeling healthy eating behaviors yourself. Children learn by observing their parents and caregivers, so make sure to prioritize nutritious foods and meals in your family's diet.
   - Involve children in meal planning, grocery shopping, and food preparation to teach them about healthy food choices and foster a positive relationship with food.

2. Balanced Diet:
   - Offer a balanced diet that includes a variety of nutrient-rich foods from all food groups. Encourage children to eat plenty of fruits, vegetables, whole grains, lean proteins, and dairy or dairy alternatives to ensure they receive essential vitamins, minerals, and other nutrients.
   - Limit the consumption of processed and junk foods high in added sugars, unhealthy fats, and sodium. Instead, provide wholesome, minimally processed foods to support overall health and well-being.

3. Regular Meals and Snacks:
   - Establish regular meal and snack times to provide structure and consistency in your child's eating routine. Aim for three balanced meals and 1-2 nutritious snacks per day to meet their energy and nutrient needs.
   - Offer a variety of healthy options at each meal and snack to encourage variety and ensure adequate nutrient intake throughout the day.

4. Portion Control:
   - Practice portion control and serve appropriate portion sizes for your child's age and appetite. Use child-sized plates, bowls, and utensils to help gauge portion sizes and prevent overeating.
   - Encourage children to listen to their hunger and fullness cues and avoid pressuring them to clean their plates or eat more than they need.

5. Hydration:

- Promote regular hydration by offering water throughout the day and encouraging children to drink water with meals and snacks. Limit the consumption of sugary beverages like soda, fruit juice, and sports drinks, which can contribute to excess calorie intake and dental cavities.
- Make water easily accessible and appealing by providing reusable water bottles and infusing water with fresh fruits or herbs for added flavor.

6. Family Meals:

- Prioritize family meals whenever possible, as they offer valuable opportunities for connection, communication, and bonding. Family meals provide a chance to model healthy eating behaviors, share positive mealtime experiences, and reinforce the importance of nutritious foods.
- Aim to create a relaxed and enjoyable atmosphere during meals, free from distractions like screens or electronic devices, to promote mindful eating and positive mealtime interactions.

7. Encourage Exploration and Variety:

- Encourage children to explore new foods and flavors and be open to trying different types of foods from a young age. Offer a wide variety of foods and expose children to diverse cuisines and cultural dishes to expand their palates and promote dietary diversity.
- Involve children in meal planning and preparation to empower them to make healthy food choices and develop a sense of ownership and autonomy over their diets.

8. Be Patient and Persistent:

- Building healthy eating habits takes time and patience, so be consistent and persistent in your efforts to promote nutritious eating habits in children. Be patient with picky eaters and continue to offer a variety of healthy foods, even if they are initially met with resistance.
- Stay positive and focus on progress rather than perfection, celebrating small victories and milestones along the way. With patience, encouragement, and consistency, children can develop lifelong healthy eating habits that support their health and well-being.

Teenagers and Nutritional Needs

Nutritional needs during the teenage years are crucial for supporting growth, development, and overall health. Adolescence is a period of rapid physical and emotional changes, making it essential to prioritize nutrient-rich foods to meet the increased demands of this life stage. Here are some important considerations for teenagers and their nutritional needs:

1. Energy Requirements:
   - During adolescence, energy requirements increase significantly to support growth spurts, physical activity, and metabolic demands. Teenagers need an adequate intake of calories to fuel their active lifestyles and support proper growth and development.

2. Protein:
   - Protein is essential for building and repairing tissues, muscles, and organs, making it especially important for teenagers who are undergoing rapid growth and development. Encourage teenagers to include lean sources of protein such as poultry, fish, beans, lentils, tofu, and dairy or dairy alternatives in their diet.

3. Calcium and Vitamin D:
   - Calcium and vitamin D are crucial for bone health and development during adolescence. Teenagers should aim to consume adequate amounts of calcium-rich foods such as dairy products, leafy green vegetables, fortified plant-based milk, and fortified foods. Vitamin D helps the body absorb calcium, so teenagers should also get regular sun exposure and consume vitamin D-fortified foods like fortified milk and cereals.

4. Iron:
   - Iron is important for teenagers, particularly adolescent girls who are at risk of iron deficiency due to menstrual blood loss. Encourage teenagers to consume iron-rich foods such as lean meats, poultry, fish, beans, lentils, tofu, fortified cereals, and dark leafy greens to support healthy blood and prevent iron deficiency anemia.

5. Whole Grains:

- Whole grains provide essential nutrients and fiber, which are important for overall health and digestion. Encourage teenagers to choose whole grain options such as whole wheat bread, brown rice, quinoa, oats, and whole grain pasta over refined grains to maximize nutrient intake and support long-term health.

6. Fruits and Vegetables:
- Fruits and vegetables are rich in vitamins, minerals, antioxidants, and fiber, making them essential components of a healthy diet for teenagers. Encourage teenagers to consume a variety of colorful fruits and vegetables to ensure they receive a wide range of nutrients and support overall health and immunity.

7. Hydration:
- Proper hydration is important for teenagers, especially those who are physically active or participating in sports. Encourage teenagers to drink plenty of water throughout the day and to avoid sugary beverages like soda, sports drinks, and energy drinks, which can contribute to excess calorie intake and dehydration.

8. Healthy Fats:
- Healthy fats are important for brain health, hormone production, and overall growth and development during adolescence. Encourage teenagers to include sources of healthy fats such as avocados, nuts, seeds, olive oil, fatty fish, and nut butters in their diet to support brain function and overall health.

9. Limit Added Sugars and Processed Foods:
- Encourage teenagers to limit their intake of added sugars and processed foods, which can contribute to excess calorie intake, weight gain, and poor health outcomes. Instead, focus on nutrient-dense foods like fruits, vegetables, whole grains, lean proteins, and healthy fats to support optimal health and well-being.

10. Balanced Meals and Snacks:
- Encourage teenagers to eat balanced meals and snacks that include a combination of carbohydrates, protein, and healthy fats to provide sustained energy and satiety throughout the day. Encourage them to

avoid skipping meals and to prioritize regular, balanced eating habits to support overall health and well-being.

Adult Nutrition: Maintaining Health and Preventing Disease

Maintaining health and preventing disease through proper nutrition is essential for adults of all ages. A balanced diet can help reduce the risk of chronic diseases, support overall well-being, and promote longevity. Here are some key considerations for adult nutrition:

1. Balanced Diet:
   - Aim for a balanced diet that includes a variety of nutrient-rich foods from all food groups. Include plenty of fruits, vegetables, whole grains, lean proteins, and healthy fats in your meals to ensure you get a wide range of essential nutrients.

2. Portion Control:
   - Practice portion control to manage calorie intake and prevent overeating. Pay attention to serving sizes and listen to your body's hunger and fullness cues to avoid consuming excess calories.

3. Limit Added Sugars and Processed Foods:
   - Minimize the consumption of foods and beverages high in added sugars, unhealthy fats, and sodium. Processed and packaged foods often contain hidden sources of added sugars and unhealthy fats, so opt for whole, minimally processed foods whenever possible.

4. Choose Healthy Fats:
   - Include sources of healthy fats in your diet, such as avocados, nuts, seeds, olive oil, and fatty fish like salmon and sardines. Healthy fats support heart health, brain function, and overall well-being.

5. Increase Fiber Intake:
   - Consume plenty of fiber-rich foods like fruits, vegetables, whole grains, legumes, nuts, and seeds. Fiber helps regulate digestion,

supports gut health, and may reduce the risk of chronic diseases like heart disease, diabetes, and certain types of cancer.

6. Hydration:
   - Stay hydrated by drinking plenty of water throughout the day. Aim to drink at least 8 glasses of water per day, or more if you're physically active or in hot weather. Limit the consumption of sugary beverages and alcohol, which can contribute to excess calorie intake and dehydration.

7. Include Lean Proteins:
   - Incorporate lean sources of protein into your meals, such as poultry, fish, beans, lentils, tofu, tempeh, and low-fat dairy products. Protein is essential for muscle maintenance, repair, and overall health.

8. Prioritize Whole Foods:
   - Choose whole, minimally processed foods over highly processed and packaged foods. Whole foods are generally higher in nutrients and fiber and lower in added sugars, unhealthy fats, and sodium.

9. Practice Mindful Eating:
   - Practice mindful eating by paying attention to your food choices, eating slowly, and savoring each bite. Be mindful of portion sizes, hunger and fullness cues, and the sensory experience of eating.

10. Be Physically Active:
   - Regular physical activity is an essential component of a healthy lifestyle. Aim for at least 150 minutes of moderate-intensity aerobic exercise or 75 minutes of vigorous-intensity aerobic exercise per week, along with muscle-strengthening activities on two or more days per week.

11. Get Regular Check-Ups:
   - Schedule regular check-ups with your healthcare provider to monitor your health status, address any concerns, and receive personalized recommendations for nutrition and lifestyle modifications.

Nutrition for Older Adults and Healthy Aging

Nutrition plays a vital role in promoting healthy aging and maintaining quality of life for older adults. As individuals age, their nutritional needs may change due to factors such as changes in metabolism, reduced appetite, and increased risk of chronic diseases. Here are some key considerations for nutrition in older adults:

1. Nutrient-Dense Foods:
- Focus on nutrient-dense foods that provide essential vitamins, minerals, fiber, and antioxidants. Incorporate a variety of colorful fruits, vegetables, whole grains, lean proteins, and healthy fats into your diet to ensure you meet your nutritional needs.

2. Protein Intake:
- Adequate protein intake is important for maintaining muscle mass, strength, and overall health in older adults. Include sources of high-quality protein such as lean meats, poultry, fish, eggs, dairy products, legumes, and tofu in your meals.

3. Fiber-Rich Foods:
- Increase your intake of fiber-rich foods like fruits, vegetables, whole grains, legumes, nuts, and seeds to support digestive health, regulate bowel movements, and reduce the risk of constipation.

4. Hydration:
- Stay hydrated by drinking plenty of fluids throughout the day, even if you don't feel thirsty. Older adults may have a decreased sensation of thirst, so it's important to drink water regularly to prevent dehydration.

5. Calcium and Vitamin D:
- Calcium and vitamin D are essential for bone health and preventing osteoporosis in older adults. Include calcium-rich foods such as dairy products, fortified plant-based milk, leafy green vegetables, and fortified foods in your diet. Get regular sun exposure and consider taking a vitamin D supplement if needed.

6. Omega-3 Fatty Acids:

- Omega-3 fatty acids have anti-inflammatory properties and may help reduce the risk of heart disease and cognitive decline in older adults. Include sources of omega-3 fatty acids such as fatty fish (salmon, mackerel, sardines), flaxseeds, chia seeds, walnuts, and algae-based supplements in your diet.

7. Limit Sodium and Processed Foods:

- Reduce your intake of sodium and processed foods, which can contribute to high blood pressure, heart disease, and other chronic conditions. Choose fresh, whole foods and limit the consumption of packaged and processed foods high in sodium, added sugars, and unhealthy fats.

8. Stay Active:

- Engage in regular physical activity to maintain muscle strength, flexibility, balance, and cardiovascular health. Aim for a combination of aerobic exercise, strength training, flexibility exercises, and balance exercises to support overall health and mobility.

9. Meal Planning and Preparation:

- Plan and prepare nutritious meals and snacks ahead of time to ensure you have healthy options readily available. Cook meals at home using fresh ingredients and incorporate a variety of flavors and textures to make eating enjoyable.

10. Socialize and Enjoy Meals:

- Share meals with family and friends whenever possible to promote social connection and enjoyment of food. Eating together can enhance appetite, improve mood, and provide opportunities for meaningful social interaction.

11. Regular Health Screenings:

- Schedule regular health screenings with your healthcare provider to monitor your nutritional status, manage chronic conditions, and address any concerns related to diet and health.

Chapter 11
Nutrition and
Physical Activity

The Synergy of Nutrition and Exercise

The synergy of nutrition and exercise is a powerful combination that promotes overall health, supports weight management, and enhances athletic performance. When paired together, proper nutrition and regular physical activity can maximize the benefits of each and lead to better health outcomes. Here's how nutrition and exercise work together synergistically:

1. Energy Balance:
- Nutrition provides the fuel necessary for physical activity, while exercise helps to expend energy. Achieving a balance between calorie intake and expenditure is essential for maintaining a healthy weight and supporting overall health.

2. Nutrient Timing:
- Consuming the right nutrients at the right times can optimize performance and recovery during exercise. Pre-workout meals or snacks provide the energy needed for exercise, while post-workout nutrition supports muscle repair and recovery.

3. Muscle Building and Repair:
- Protein is essential for building and repairing muscles, which is crucial for athletes and individuals engaging in regular exercise. Consuming adequate protein from sources like lean meats, poultry, fish, dairy, eggs, legumes, and plant-based protein sources can support muscle growth and repair.

4. Hydration:
- Proper hydration is essential for optimizing exercise performance and supporting overall health. Water helps regulate body temperature, transport nutrients, and remove waste products from the body. Staying hydrated before, during, and after exercise is critical for maintaining optimal hydration levels.

5. Macronutrient Balance:
- Carbohydrates provide the primary source of energy for exercise, while fats serve as an additional fuel source, especially during prolonged endurance activities. Balancing carbohydrate and fat intake

can optimize energy availability for exercise while supporting overall health.

6. Micronutrient Support:

- Vitamins and minerals play important roles in energy metabolism, muscle function, and recovery. Consuming a varied and balanced diet rich in fruits, vegetables, whole grains, lean proteins, and healthy fats can provide essential vitamins and minerals needed for optimal health and exercise performance.

7. Weight Management:

- Regular physical activity helps to burn calories and maintain a healthy weight, while proper nutrition supports weight management by providing the nutrients needed for energy and metabolism. Combining a balanced diet with regular exercise can help achieve and maintain a healthy body weight.

8. Bone Health:

- Weight-bearing exercises like walking, running, and strength training can help build and maintain bone density, reducing the risk of osteoporosis and fractures. Consuming adequate calcium and vitamin D through diet or supplements can further support bone health.

9. Mental Health Benefits:

- Both nutrition and exercise have been shown to have positive effects on mental health and well-being. Regular physical activity can reduce stress, anxiety, and depression, while proper nutrition supports brain function and mood regulation.

10. Long-Term Health:

- The combination of nutrition and exercise has long-term benefits for overall health and disease prevention. Regular physical activity and a balanced diet can reduce the risk of chronic diseases such as heart disease, diabetes, obesity, and certain cancers.

Pre- and Post-Workout Nutrition

Pre- and post-workout nutrition are crucial components of an effective exercise routine. Properly fueling your body before and after exercise can enhance performance, support muscle growth and repair, and optimize recovery. Here's what you need to know about pre- and post-workout nutrition:

Pre-Workout Nutrition:

1. **Timing:** Aim to eat a balanced meal or snack containing carbohydrates, protein, and a small amount of healthy fats 1-3 hours before your workout. This timing allows for digestion and absorption of nutrients to provide energy during exercise.

2. **Carbohydrates:** Carbohydrates are the body's primary source of energy during exercise. Choose easily digestible carbohydrates such as fruits, whole grains, or low-fiber snacks like rice cakes or pretzels to provide quick energy.

3. **Protein:** Including a moderate amount of protein in your pre-workout meal or snack can help support muscle repair and growth. Choose lean protein sources such as chicken, turkey, fish, tofu, or Greek yogurt.

4. **Hydration:** Drink plenty of water leading up to your workout to ensure proper hydration. Consider consuming a small amount of water or a sports drink 30-60 minutes before exercise to help maintain hydration levels during your workout.

5. **Avoid High-Fat and High-Fiber Foods:** Avoid consuming high-fat or high-fiber foods close to your workout, as they can cause digestive discomfort and slow digestion, leading to discomfort during exercise.

6. **Sample Pre-Workout Meals or Snacks:**
   - Whole grain toast with almond butter and sliced banana
   - Greek yogurt with berries and a drizzle of honey
   - Oatmeal topped with nuts and diced fruit
   - Whole grain cereal with milk or a milk alternative
   - Turkey and cheese sandwich on whole wheat bread

Post-Workout Nutrition:

1. **Timing:** Consume a combination of carbohydrates and protein within 30-60 minutes after your workout to replenish glycogen stores, support muscle recovery, and promote muscle protein synthesis.

2. **Carbohydrates:** Consuming carbohydrates after exercise helps replenish glycogen stores and provides energy for recovery. Choose complex carbohydrates such as whole grains, fruits, vegetables, or starchy vegetables like sweet potatoes or squash.

3. **Protein:** Protein is essential for muscle repair and growth after exercise. Include a source of lean protein such as chicken, fish, tofu, eggs, or a protein shake to provide amino acids necessary for muscle recovery.

4. **Hydration:** Rehydrate by drinking water or a sports drink after your workout to replace fluids lost through sweat. Aim to drink enough fluid to replenish any losses during exercise.

5. **Electrolytes:** If you engaged in intense or prolonged exercise, consider consuming foods or beverages containing electrolytes such as sodium and potassium to help replace losses and restore electrolyte balance.

6. **Sample Post-Workout Meals or Snacks:**
   - Grilled chicken salad with mixed greens, vegetables, and quinoa
   - Smoothie made with protein powder, spinach, banana, and almond milk
   - Greek yogurt parfait with granola and mixed berries
   - Whole grain wrap with turkey, avocado, and vegetables
   - Cottage cheese with pineapple chunks and whole grain crackers

Fueling for Endurance vs. Strength Training

Fueling for endurance training and strength training requires different nutritional strategies to support the specific demands of each type of exercise. Here's how to fuel effectively for endurance vs. strength training:

Fueling for Endurance Training:

1. **Carbohydrates:** Endurance training requires sustained energy, so carbohydrates are essential for fueling long-duration workouts. Prioritize complex carbohydrates such as whole grains, fruits, vegetables, and legumes to provide a steady source of energy and support glycogen stores.

2. **Timing:** Consume a carbohydrate-rich meal or snack 2-3 hours before your endurance workout to provide sustained energy. Consider including easily digestible carbohydrates closer to your workout, such as a piece of fruit or energy gel, 30-60 minutes before exercise to top up glycogen stores.

3. **Hydration:** Proper hydration is crucial for endurance training to maintain performance and prevent dehydration. Drink plenty of water throughout the day leading up to your workout and consider consuming a sports drink or electrolyte beverage during longer workouts to replenish electrolytes lost through sweat.

4. **Protein:** While carbohydrates are the primary focus for endurance training, don't neglect protein. Including a small amount of protein with your pre-workout meal or snack can help support muscle repair and prevent muscle breakdown during prolonged exercise.

5. **Electrolytes:** During longer endurance workouts, especially in hot or humid conditions, consider consuming foods or beverages containing electrolytes such as sodium and potassium to help maintain electrolyte balance and prevent cramping.

Fueling for Strength Training:

1. **Protein:** Protein is essential for muscle repair and growth, making it a key component of fueling for strength training. Consume a source of high-quality protein such as lean meats, poultry, fish, eggs, dairy

products, or plant-based protein sources with each meal and snack throughout the day.

2. **Carbohydrates:** While carbohydrates are important for providing energy during strength training, they are not as critical as they are for endurance exercise. Focus on consuming complex carbohydrates to support overall energy levels and glycogen replenishment, but prioritize protein intake for muscle recovery.

3. **Timing:** Aim to consume a balanced meal or snack containing protein and carbohydrates 1-2 hours before your strength training session to provide energy and support muscle repair. After your workout, prioritize protein intake to promote muscle recovery and repair.

4. **Hydration:** Proper hydration is important for strength training to support muscle function, performance, and recovery. Drink water throughout the day leading up to your workout and continue to hydrate during and after your strength training session.

5. **Post-Workout Nutrition:** After strength training, prioritize protein intake to support muscle repair and growth. Consuming a source of protein within 30-60 minutes after your workout, along with carbohydrates to replenish glycogen stores, can enhance muscle recovery and adaptation.

6. **Supplementation:** Some strength athletes may benefit from supplementation with creatine monohydrate, which has been shown to improve strength, power, and muscle mass when combined with resistance training.

Hydration and Exercise Performance

Hydration is crucial for exercise performance as it plays a significant role in regulating body temperature, maintaining fluid balance, transporting nutrients, and supporting overall physiological function. Proper hydration before, during, and after exercise can help optimize performance, delay fatigue, and reduce the risk of dehydration-related complications. Here's how hydration impacts exercise performance:

1. Pre-Exercise Hydration:
   - Begin your workout adequately hydrated by drinking water
throughout the day leading up to your exercise session. Aim to consume
about 16-20 ounces of water 2-3 hours before exercise to ensure proper
hydration status.

2. During-Exercise Hydration:
   - Drink fluids during exercise to replace fluids lost through sweating
and maintain hydration levels. The amount of fluid needed depends on
factors such as exercise intensity, duration, environmental conditions,
and individual sweat rates.
   - For shorter workouts (less than 60 minutes), water is generally
sufficient for maintaining hydration. Sip water regularly during your
workout to stay hydrated.
   - For longer workouts or high-intensity exercise lasting more than 60
minutes, consider consuming a sports drink or electrolyte beverage to
replenish electrolytes lost through sweat and provide additional
carbohydrates for energy.
   - Monitor your hydration status during exercise by paying attention to
thirst, urine color (pale yellow is ideal), and sweat rate. Adjust your
fluid intake accordingly to maintain proper hydration levels.

3. Post-Exercise Hydration:
   - Rehydrate after exercise by drinking fluids to replace fluids lost
during the workout. Aim to consume about 16-24 ounces of fluid for
every pound of body weight lost during exercise.
   - Include electrolytes in your post-exercise hydration strategy to
replenish sodium, potassium, and other electrolytes lost through sweat.
Consuming a sports drink or electrolyte beverage can help restore
electrolyte balance and support hydration.

4. Electrolyte Balance:
   - Electrolytes such as sodium, potassium, chloride, and magnesium
are essential for maintaining fluid balance, nerve function, muscle
contraction, and overall hydration status. During prolonged or intense
exercise, electrolyte losses through sweat can contribute to
dehydration and electrolyte imbalances.

- Consuming foods or beverages containing electrolytes, such as sports drinks, electrolyte tablets, or salty snacks, can help replace electrolytes lost during exercise and maintain proper electrolyte balance.

5. Individual Hydration Needs:
- Hydration needs vary depending on factors such as body weight, sweat rate, exercise intensity, duration, and environmental conditions. It's essential to listen to your body and adjust your fluid intake based on your individual hydration needs and preferences.

6. Signs of Dehydration:
- Recognize the signs and symptoms of dehydration, including thirst, dry mouth, dark urine, fatigue, headache, dizziness, and decreased performance. Dehydration can impair exercise performance, increase the risk of heat-related illnesses, and negatively impact overall health and well-being.

7. Hydration Strategies:
- Develop a hydration plan that works for you based on your individual needs, preferences, and exercise routine. Experiment with different fluids, timing, and strategies to find what works best for maintaining optimal hydration and performance.

Creating Sustainable Fitness and Nutrition Habits

Creating sustainable fitness and nutrition habits is essential for long-term health and well-being. Instead of short-term fixes or fad diets, focus on making gradual, lasting changes to your lifestyle that you can maintain over time. Here are some tips for creating sustainable fitness and nutrition habits:

1. Set Realistic Goals:
- Set achievable goals that are specific, measurable, attainable, relevant, and time-bound (SMART). Start with small, realistic goals and gradually increase the intensity or duration as you progress.

2. Make Gradual Changes:

- Focus on making small, sustainable changes to your fitness and
nutrition habits over time. Rather than trying to overhaul your entire
lifestyle overnight, start by incorporating one healthy habit at a time
and gradually build upon your progress.

3. Find Activities You Enjoy:
- Choose physical activities and exercises that you enjoy and look
forward to doing. Whether it's walking, running, cycling, swimming,
dancing, or playing sports, find activities that fit your interests,
preferences, and lifestyle.

4. Prioritize Consistency Over Perfection:
- Consistency is key to long-term success. Aim for consistency in your
fitness and nutrition habits rather than striving for perfection.
Remember that small, consistent efforts add up over time and lead to
significant progress.

5. Focus on Whole Foods:
- Prioritize whole, minimally processed foods in your diet, such as
fruits, vegetables, whole grains, lean proteins, and healthy fats. Focus
on nourishing your body with nutrient-dense foods that provide
essential vitamins, minerals, fiber, and antioxidants.

6. Practice Portion Control:
- Pay attention to portion sizes and listen to your body's hunger and
fullness cues. Practice mindful eating by savoring each bite, eating
slowly, and paying attention to the sensations of hunger and
satisfaction.

7. Stay Hydrated:
- Drink plenty of water throughout the day to stay hydrated and
support overall health. Carry a reusable water bottle with you and sip
water regularly to maintain hydration levels, especially during exercise
or in hot weather.

8. Plan and Prepare Meals:
- Plan and prepare meals ahead of time to ensure you have healthy
options readily available. Batch cook meals, pack lunches, and snacks,

and stock your kitchen with nutritious foods to make healthy eating more convenient and accessible.

9. Practice Self-Care:
 - Prioritize self-care and stress management as part of your overall health and wellness routine. Incorporate activities such as meditation, yoga, deep breathing exercises, or spending time outdoors to reduce stress and promote relaxation.

10. Seek Support and Accountability:
 - Surround yourself with a supportive network of friends, family, or fitness buddies who share similar health and wellness goals. Having a support system can provide encouragement, motivation, and accountability on your journey.

11. Celebrate Your Progress:
 - Celebrate your achievements and progress along the way, no matter how small. Acknowledge your efforts and successes, and use them as motivation to keep moving forward on your journey towards better health and well-being.

Chapter 12
Dietary Supplements: Pros and Cons

Understanding Dietary Supplements

Dietary supplements are products intended to supplement the diet and provide essential nutrients that may be lacking in one's regular diet. While supplements can be beneficial in certain situations, it's essential to understand their role, benefits, and potential drawbacks. Here's an overview of dietary supplements:

1. Types of Dietary Supplements:
  - **Vitamins:** These are micronutrients essential for various bodily functions, including metabolism, immune function, and overall health. Common vitamins include vitamin C, vitamin D, vitamin B complex, and vitamin E.
  - **Minerals:** Minerals are essential for maintaining healthy bones, teeth, muscles, and nerve function. Examples include calcium, magnesium, iron, zinc, and potassium.
  - **Herbal Supplements:** These are products made from plants or plant extracts and are often used for their purported health benefits. Examples include ginkgo biloba, echinacea, garlic, and turmeric.
  - **Protein Powders:** These supplements provide concentrated sources of protein, typically derived from whey, casein, soy, pea, or rice protein. They are commonly used by athletes and individuals looking to increase protein intake.
  - **Omega-3 Fatty Acids:** Omega-3 supplements contain essential fatty acids that are important for heart health, brain function, and inflammation regulation. They are commonly derived from fish oil, krill oil, or algae oil.
  - **Probiotics:** These are live microorganisms that are beneficial for gut health and digestion. Probiotic supplements contain strains of bacteria or yeast intended to promote a healthy gut microbiome.
  - **Multivitamins:** Multivitamin supplements contain a combination of vitamins and minerals to help fill nutrient gaps in the diet.

2. Pros of Dietary Supplements:
  - **Nutrient Deficiency Prevention:** Supplements can help prevent or address nutrient deficiencies, especially in individuals with restricted diets, certain medical conditions, or increased nutrient needs (e.g., pregnant women, athletes).

- **Convenience:** Supplements provide a convenient way to ensure adequate nutrient intake, particularly for busy individuals who may struggle to meet their nutritional needs through diet alone.
- **Targeted Support:** Certain supplements may offer targeted support for specific health concerns or goals, such as bone health, immune support, joint health, or cognitive function.
- **Athletic Performance:** Some supplements, such as protein powders, creatine, and branched-chain amino acids (BCAAs), are popular among athletes and fitness enthusiasts to support muscle growth, recovery, and performance.

3. Cons of Dietary Supplements:

- **Lack of Regulation:** The supplement industry is not as tightly regulated as the pharmaceutical industry, leading to concerns about product safety, quality, and efficacy. Some supplements may contain contaminants, impurities, or inaccurate labeling.
- **Potential Side Effects:** Certain supplements may cause adverse effects, interactions with medications, or allergic reactions in susceptible individuals. It's essential to consult with a healthcare provider before starting any new supplement regimen, especially if you have underlying health conditions or take medications.
- **Cost:** Regular use of dietary supplements can be costly, especially if multiple supplements are taken regularly. It's important to consider the financial implications and whether the benefits justify the expense.
- **Nutrient Overload:** Taking excessive amounts of certain vitamins or minerals through supplements can lead to nutrient imbalances or toxicity. It's important to follow recommended dosages and avoid megadoses unless advised by a healthcare professional.

4. Considerations for Supplement Use:

- **Consult with Healthcare Provider:** Before starting any new supplement regimen, consult with a qualified healthcare provider, such as a physician, registered dietitian, or pharmacist. They can help assess your individual needs, recommend appropriate supplements, and ensure safety and efficacy.
- **Choose Reputable Brands:** Select supplements from reputable brands that adhere to good manufacturing practices (GMP) and have undergone third-party testing for quality, purity, and potency.
- **Read Labels Carefully:** Pay close attention to supplement labels, including the ingredient list, dosage recommendations, and any

potential warnings or contraindications. Avoid supplements with unnecessary additives, fillers, or proprietary blends.

- **Use Supplements as a Complement:** Dietary supplements should complement, not replace, a healthy and balanced diet. Focus on obtaining nutrients from whole foods whenever possible, and use supplements as a backup or to address specific deficiencies or needs.

Commonly Used Vitamins and Minerals

Commonly used vitamins and minerals are essential nutrients that play crucial roles in maintaining overall health and well-being. While it's best to obtain these nutrients through a balanced diet, some individuals may choose to supplement their intake to address deficiencies or support specific health goals. Here are some of the most commonly used vitamins and minerals:

1. Vitamin C (Ascorbic Acid):
   - **Function:** Vitamin C is a powerful antioxidant that supports immune function, collagen synthesis, wound healing, and iron absorption.
   - **Food Sources:** Citrus fruits (oranges, lemons, grapefruits), strawberries, kiwi, bell peppers, broccoli, kale, and tomatoes.
   - **Supplement Use:** Vitamin C supplements are commonly used to support immune health, especially during cold and flu season, and may be taken in higher doses for antioxidant support.

2. Vitamin D:
   - **Function:** Vitamin D is essential for bone health, calcium absorption, immune function, and overall health.
   - **Food Sources:** Fatty fish (salmon, mackerel, sardines), fortified dairy products, fortified cereals, egg yolks, and sunlight exposure (UVB rays trigger vitamin D synthesis in the skin).
   - **Supplement Use:** Many people have insufficient vitamin D levels, especially those with limited sun exposure or living in northern latitudes. Vitamin D supplements may be recommended to maintain adequate levels, particularly during the winter months.

3. Vitamin B12 (Cobalamin):

- **Function:** Vitamin B12 is essential for nerve function, red blood cell production, DNA synthesis, and energy metabolism.
- **Food Sources:** Animal products (meat, fish, poultry, dairy products, eggs), fortified plant-based foods (nutritional yeast, fortified cereals, fortified plant milks).
- **Supplement Use:** Vitamin B12 deficiency is common among vegetarians, vegans, and older adults. B12 supplements may be necessary for those who do not consume adequate dietary sources or have absorption issues.

4. Iron:

- **Function:** Iron is essential for oxygen transport, energy production, and overall metabolism.
- **Food Sources:** Red meat, poultry, fish, lentils, beans, tofu, fortified cereals, spinach, and other leafy greens.
- **Supplement Use:** Iron deficiency is one of the most common nutrient deficiencies worldwide, especially among menstruating individuals, pregnant women, and vegetarians/vegans. Iron supplements may be necessary to treat or prevent deficiency, but should be used under medical supervision due to the risk of iron overload.

5. Calcium:

- **Function:** Calcium is crucial for bone and teeth health, muscle function, nerve transmission, and blood clotting.
- **Food Sources:** Dairy products (milk, yogurt, cheese), fortified plant-based milks, leafy greens (kale, collard greens), tofu, almonds, and fortified foods.
- **Supplement Use:** Calcium supplements may be recommended for individuals who do not consume enough dietary calcium, especially those at risk of osteoporosis or bone fractures.

6. Magnesium:

- **Function:** Magnesium is involved in over 300 biochemical reactions in the body, including energy production, muscle function, nerve transmission, and bone health.
- **Food Sources:** Nuts, seeds, whole grains, leafy greens, legumes, tofu, avocado, bananas, and dark chocolate.

  - **Supplement Use:** Magnesium supplements may be used to support overall health and well-being, especially for individuals with inadequate dietary intake or certain health conditions.

7. Omega-3 Fatty Acids:
  - **Function:** Omega-3 fatty acids are essential fats that support heart health, brain function, eye health, and inflammation regulation.
  - **Food Sources:** Fatty fish (salmon, mackerel, sardines), flaxseeds, chia seeds, walnuts, hemp seeds, and algae oil.
  - **Supplement Use:** Omega-3 supplements, such as fish oil or algae oil, may be recommended for individuals who do not consume enough fatty fish or plant-based sources of omega-3s.

8. Zinc:
  - **Function:** Zinc is essential for immune function, wound healing, DNA synthesis, and cell division.
  - **Food Sources:** Red meat, poultry, seafood, beans, nuts, seeds, whole grains, dairy products, and fortified cereals.
  - **Supplement Use:** Zinc supplements may be used to support immune health, especially during times of increased susceptibility to infections.

Herbal Supplements and Their Considerations

Herbal supplements are products made from plants or plant extracts that are consumed for their purported health benefits. While herbal supplements have been used for centuries in traditional medicine practices, it's important to approach their use with caution and understanding. Here are some considerations regarding herbal supplements:

1. Types of Herbal Supplements:
  - **Echinacea:** Often used to support immune function and reduce the severity and duration of colds and respiratory infections.
  - **Ginkgo Biloba:** Claimed to improve memory, cognitive function, and circulation, and may be used for conditions such as dementia and Alzheimer's disease.

- **Turmeric (Curcumin):** Known for its anti-inflammatory properties and may be used to reduce inflammation, joint pain, and symptoms of arthritis.
- **Garlic:** Used to support heart health, lower cholesterol levels, and boost immune function.
- **Ginseng:** Claimed to increase energy, reduce stress, improve mental clarity, and enhance physical performance.
- **Valerian Root:** Often used as a natural remedy for insomnia, anxiety, and stress management.
- **St. John's Wort:** Used to treat symptoms of depression, anxiety, and mood disorders.

2. Potential Benefits:

- **Natural Remedies:** Herbal supplements are often perceived as natural alternatives to conventional medications and may be used to address various health concerns.
- **Traditional Medicine:** Many herbal supplements have been used for centuries in traditional medicine practices, and some may have evidence supporting their efficacy for specific conditions.

3. Considerations:

- **Limited Regulation:** Herbal supplements are not as tightly regulated as pharmaceutical drugs, and there may be variations in quality, purity, and potency among different products. It's essential to choose reputable brands that adhere to good manufacturing practices (GMP) and have undergone third-party testing for quality and safety.
- **Potential Side Effects:** Herbal supplements can cause side effects, adverse reactions, and interactions with medications. It's important to research potential risks and consult with a healthcare professional before starting any new herbal supplement regimen, especially if you have underlying health conditions or take medications.
- **Efficacy:** While some herbal supplements have research supporting their efficacy for specific health conditions, others may lack scientific evidence or have conflicting results. It's essential to critically evaluate the available research and approach herbal supplements with a healthy skepticism.
- **Dosage and Safety:** Herbal supplements may have recommended dosages, contraindications, and precautions that should be followed to ensure safety and efficacy. It's important to read product labels

carefully, follow dosage instructions, and be aware of any warnings or cautions associated with specific herbs.

- **Interactions with Medications:** Herbal supplements can interact with prescription medications, over-the-counter drugs, and other supplements, potentially affecting their efficacy or safety. It's important to disclose all supplements you are taking to your healthcare provider to avoid potential interactions.

- **Pregnancy and Lactation:** Some herbal supplements may not be safe during pregnancy or breastfeeding and may pose risks to maternal and fetal health. Pregnant or lactating individuals should consult with a healthcare professional before using herbal supplements.

4. Personalization and Individual Response:

- Herbal supplements may have varying effects on different individuals, and responses can vary based on factors such as age, gender, health status, genetics, and lifestyle. What works for one person may not work for another, so it's essential to pay attention to your body's response and adjust your supplement regimen accordingly.

5. Quality and Source:

- Choose herbal supplements from reputable brands that prioritize quality, purity, and transparency. Look for products that have undergone third-party testing for quality assurance and are free from contaminants, fillers, and unnecessary additives.

Risks and Benefits of Supplement Use

The use of dietary supplements can offer both potential benefits and risks, depending on various factors such as individual health status, the specific supplement, dosage, and duration of use. Here's an overview of the risks and benefits associated with supplement use:

Benefits of Supplement Use:

1. **Addressing Nutrient Deficiencies:** Supplements can help fill nutrient gaps in the diet, especially for individuals who have limited access to certain foods, follow restrictive diets (e.g., vegan or

vegetarian), or have increased nutrient needs (e.g., pregnant women, athletes).

2. **Supporting Specific Health Goals:** Certain supplements may offer targeted support for specific health concerns or goals, such as immune support, bone health, heart health, cognitive function, or athletic performance.

3. **Convenience and Accessibility:** Supplements provide a convenient and accessible way to obtain essential nutrients, especially for individuals with busy lifestyles who may struggle to meet their nutritional needs through diet alone.

4. **Prevention and Management of Health Conditions:** Some supplements may play a role in preventing or managing certain health conditions, such as vitamin D for bone health, omega-3 fatty acids for heart health, or probiotics for gut health.

5. **Enhancing Athletic Performance:** Certain supplements, such as protein powders, creatine, and branched-chain amino acids (BCAAs), are popular among athletes and fitness enthusiasts to support muscle growth, recovery, and performance.

Risks of Supplement Use:

1. **Potential for Harm:** Supplements are not risk-free, and excessive or inappropriate use can lead to adverse effects, interactions with medications, nutrient imbalances, or toxicity. Certain supplements may pose risks, especially when taken in high doses or for prolonged periods.

2. **Lack of Regulation:** The supplement industry is not as tightly regulated as the pharmaceutical industry, leading to concerns about product safety, quality, purity, and accuracy of labeling. Some supplements may contain contaminants, impurities, or undisclosed ingredients.

3. **False Claims and Misinformation:** There is often a lack of scientific evidence supporting the efficacy and safety of many dietary

supplements, and some products may make exaggerated claims or rely on anecdotal evidence rather than rigorous scientific research.

4. **Interactions with Medications:** Supplements can interact with prescription medications, over-the-counter drugs, and other supplements, potentially affecting their efficacy or safety. It's essential to consult with a healthcare professional before starting any new supplement regimen, especially if you take medications or have underlying health conditions.

5. **Financial Cost:** Regular use of dietary supplements can be costly, especially if multiple supplements are taken regularly. It's important to consider the financial implications and whether the benefits justify the expense.

6. **Potential for Dependency:** Relying too heavily on supplements to meet nutritional needs can lead to a dependency on these products and may detract from the importance of obtaining nutrients from whole foods.

Consulting with Healthcare Professionals about Supplements

Consulting with healthcare professionals about supplements is essential to ensure their safe and effective use, as well as to minimize potential risks. Here's why it's important to seek guidance from healthcare professionals before starting any new supplement regimen:

1. **Individualized Assessment:**
   - Healthcare professionals can conduct an individualized assessment of your health status, medical history, dietary habits, and lifestyle factors to determine whether supplements are necessary and appropriate for you.

2. **Identification of Nutrient Deficiencies:**
   - Healthcare professionals can identify potential nutrient deficiencies through blood tests and other diagnostic assessments. Based on these

findings, they can recommend specific supplements to address any deficiencies in your diet.

3. Evaluation of Health Goals:

- Healthcare professionals can help you identify and prioritize your health goals and determine whether supplements may be beneficial in achieving those goals. They can provide personalized recommendations based on your unique needs and objectives.

4. Consideration of Medication Interactions:

- Healthcare professionals can evaluate potential interactions between supplements and medications you may be taking. Certain supplements can interact with prescription medications, affecting their efficacy or safety. Healthcare professionals can advise you on potential interactions and adjustments to your medication regimen if necessary.

5. Assessment of Supplement Quality and Safety:

- Healthcare professionals can provide guidance on selecting reputable brands and high-quality supplements that meet safety and efficacy standards. They can recommend products that have undergone third-party testing for purity, potency, and quality assurance.

6. Monitoring for Adverse Effects:

- Healthcare professionals can monitor your response to supplements and assess for any adverse effects or reactions. They can help you recognize signs of toxicity or intolerance and make adjustments to your supplement regimen as needed.

7. Guidance on Dosage and Timing:

- Healthcare professionals can provide recommendations on the appropriate dosage, frequency, and timing of supplement intake based on your individual needs and health goals. They can help you avoid excessive intake or improper use of supplements.

8. Education and Empowerment:

- Healthcare professionals can educate you about the potential benefits and risks of supplement use, empowering you to make informed decisions about your health. They can provide evidence-based information and help you distinguish between fact and fiction when it comes to supplement claims.

9. Long-Term Monitoring and Follow-Up:
   - Healthcare professionals can monitor your progress over time and provide ongoing support and guidance regarding your supplement regimen. They can adjust recommendations as needed based on changes in your health status, goals, or lifestyle factors.

10. Collaboration and Holistic Care:
   - By consulting with healthcare professionals about supplement use, you can benefit from a collaborative and holistic approach to your health and wellness. Healthcare professionals can work together with you to develop a comprehensive plan that addresses your nutritional needs, health goals, and overall well-being.

Chapter 13
Nutrition and Weight Management

The Connection Between Diet and Weight

The connection between diet and weight is central to understanding nutrition and weight management. Here's an overview of how diet influences weight:

1. Caloric Balance:
   - Weight management ultimately comes down to the balance between calories consumed and calories expended. If you consume more calories than your body needs for energy, you'll likely gain weight. Conversely, if you consume fewer calories than your body needs, you'll likely lose weight.

2. Macronutrient Composition:
   - The macronutrient composition of your diet (carbohydrates, proteins, and fats) plays a significant role in weight management. Each macronutrient has a different effect on hunger, satiety, and metabolism.
   - **Carbohydrates:** Carbohydrates are the body's primary source of energy. Consuming too many refined carbohydrates (e.g., sugary foods, white bread, pastries) can lead to spikes in blood sugar levels and increased hunger, potentially contributing to weight gain.
   - **Proteins:** Protein is essential for muscle repair, growth, and satiety. Including adequate protein in your diet can help you feel full and satisfied, reducing overall calorie intake and supporting weight management.
   - **Fats:** Dietary fats are important for hormone production, cell membrane structure, and nutrient absorption. Healthy fats, such as those found in nuts, seeds, avocados, and fatty fish, can promote satiety and support weight management when consumed in moderation.

3. Nutrient Density:
   - Choosing nutrient-dense foods, such as fruits, vegetables, whole grains, lean proteins, and healthy fats, can help you meet your nutritional needs while managing your weight. These foods are typically lower in calories and higher in essential nutrients, fiber, and antioxidants, making them ideal choices for weight management.

4. Portion Control:
  - Paying attention to portion sizes is crucial for managing calorie intake and controlling weight. Even healthy foods can contribute to weight gain if consumed in excessive amounts. Using smaller plates, measuring portions, and practicing mindful eating can help you maintain appropriate portion sizes.

5. Food Choices and Quality:
  - The types of foods you choose to eat can have a significant impact on your weight. Whole, minimally processed foods are generally more satisfying and nutrient-dense than highly processed, calorie-dense foods. Prioritizing whole foods such as fruits, vegetables, whole grains, lean proteins, and healthy fats can support weight management and overall health.

6. Mindful Eating:
  - Mindful eating involves paying attention to hunger and fullness cues, eating slowly, and savoring each bite. By tuning into your body's natural hunger and satiety signals, you can avoid overeating and make more mindful food choices, which can support weight management.

7. Hydration:
  - Staying hydrated is essential for overall health and can support weight management. Drinking water before meals can help you feel fuller and may lead to consuming fewer calories. Choosing water or other low-calorie beverages over sugary drinks can also help reduce overall calorie intake.

8. Physical Activity:
  - While diet plays a significant role in weight management, physical activity is also crucial. Regular exercise helps burn calories, build muscle mass, and improve metabolic health, all of which contribute to weight management. Combining a healthy diet with regular physical activity is the most effective approach for achieving and maintaining a healthy weight.

Healthy Approaches to Weight Loss

When it comes to weight loss, adopting healthy and sustainable approaches is key to long-term success. Here are some healthy approaches to weight loss:

1. Set Realistic Goals:
   - Set achievable and realistic weight loss goals based on your individual circumstances, such as your current weight, health status, lifestyle, and personal preferences. Aim for gradual and steady progress rather than rapid weight loss, which is often unsustainable and can lead to regain.

2. Focus on Nutrition:
   - Prioritize nutrient-dense, whole foods in your diet, such as fruits, vegetables, whole grains, lean proteins, and healthy fats. These foods are rich in vitamins, minerals, fiber, and antioxidants, which support overall health and satiety.
   - Reduce your intake of processed and high-calorie foods, such as sugary snacks, refined carbohydrates, fried foods, and sugary beverages, which can contribute to weight gain and poor health outcomes.

3. Practice Portion Control:
   - Pay attention to portion sizes and avoid oversized servings, which can lead to excess calorie intake. Use smaller plates, bowls, and utensils to help control portion sizes and prevent overeating.
   - Listen to your body's hunger and fullness cues, and stop eating when you feel satisfied rather than overly full.

4. Monitor Your Intake:
   - Keep track of your food intake using a food diary, journal, or mobile app. Recording what you eat and drink can help you become more aware of your eating habits, identify areas for improvement, and make healthier choices.
   - Be mindful of mindless eating behaviors, such as eating in front of the TV or computer, snacking out of boredom or stress, and eating straight from the package. Instead, practice mindful eating by focusing on your meals and savoring each bite.

5. Stay Hydrated:

- Drink plenty of water throughout the day to stay hydrated and support weight loss. Sometimes, feelings of hunger can be mistaken for thirst. Drinking water before meals can also help you feel fuller and consume fewer calories.

- Limit your intake of sugary beverages, such as soda, juice, and energy drinks, which are high in calories and provide little nutritional value.

6. Be Physically Active:

- Incorporate regular physical activity into your routine to support weight loss and overall health. Aim for a combination of cardiovascular exercise, strength training, and flexibility exercises.

- Find activities that you enjoy and can stick with long term, whether it's walking, jogging, swimming, cycling, dancing, or group fitness classes. Consistency is key, so aim for at least 150 minutes of moderate-intensity exercise or 75 minutes of vigorous-intensity exercise per week.

7. Seek Support:

- Surround yourself with a supportive network of friends, family members, or professionals who can encourage and motivate you on your weight loss journey.

- Consider joining a weight loss support group, working with a registered dietitian or nutritionist, or seeking guidance from a healthcare professional to develop a personalized weight loss plan tailored to your needs and goals.

8. Practice Self-Compassion:

- Be kind to yourself and practice self-compassion throughout your weight loss journey. Understand that setbacks and challenges are normal, and focus on progress rather than perfection.

- Celebrate your achievements, no matter how small, and remind yourself of the positive changes you're making to improve your health and well-being.

Understanding Body Mass Index (BMI)

Understanding Body Mass Index (BMI) is crucial in assessing weight status and understanding its implications for overall health. Here's an overview of BMI:

1. What is BMI?
   - Body Mass Index (BMI) is a measure of body fat based on an individual's weight and height. It is calculated by dividing weight in kilograms by the square of height in meters (BMI = weight / height^2).
   - BMI provides a rough estimate of body fatness and is commonly used to categorize individuals into weight status categories, such as underweight, normal weight, overweight, and obesity.

2. BMI Categories:
   - **Underweight:** BMI less than 18.5
   - **Normal Weight:** BMI 18.5 to 24.9
   - **Overweight:** BMI 25 to 29.9
   - **Obesity (Class I):** BMI 30 to 34.9
   - **Obesity (Class II):** BMI 35 to 39.9
   - **Obesity (Class III):** BMI 40 or higher

3. Interpretation of BMI:
   - BMI is used as a screening tool to assess weight status and identify individuals who may be at risk for weight-related health problems.
   - While BMI is a useful population-level measure, it does not directly measure body fat percentage or distribution. Therefore, it may not accurately reflect body composition in individuals with high muscle mass or certain ethnic groups.
   - BMI categories serve as general guidelines, but individual health risks can vary based on factors such as age, sex, muscle mass, bone density, and distribution of body fat.

4. Health Implications:
   - BMI is associated with various health outcomes, including the risk of chronic diseases such as heart disease, type 2 diabetes, hypertension, stroke, certain cancers, and overall mortality.
   - Individuals with a BMI in the overweight or obese range are at higher risk for weight-related health problems, while those with a BMI in the underweight range may be at risk for nutrient deficiencies, weakened immune function, and other health issues.

5. Limitations of BMI:
- BMI has several limitations and may not provide a comprehensive assessment of an individual's health status or risk factors.
- BMI does not account for differences in body composition, such as muscle mass versus fat mass, which can influence health outcomes. For example, athletes and individuals with high muscle mass may have a higher BMI but lower body fat percentage and may not be at increased risk for health problems.
- BMI does not consider factors such as waist circumference, body shape, distribution of fat, or metabolic health, which can affect health risks independently of BMI.

6. Additional Considerations:
- While BMI is a valuable tool for assessing weight status and health risks at the population level, it should be interpreted in conjunction with other measures and clinical assessments.
- Healthcare professionals may use BMI along with other indicators, such as waist circumference, body composition analysis, medical history, and lifestyle factors, to assess overall health and develop personalized recommendations for weight management and health promotion.

Overcoming Challenges in Weight Management

Overcoming challenges in weight management requires a multifaceted approach that addresses various factors influencing eating habits, physical activity, and overall lifestyle. Here are some common challenges in weight management and strategies to overcome them:

1. Unrealistic Expectations:
- Challenge: Many individuals have unrealistic expectations about the rate of weight loss and the effort required to achieve and maintain a healthy weight.
- Strategy: Set realistic and achievable goals based on your individual circumstances, preferences, and lifestyle. Focus on making gradual and sustainable changes rather than pursuing rapid weight loss or drastic measures.

2. Emotional Eating:

- Challenge: Emotional eating, or eating in response to emotions such as stress, boredom, sadness, or anxiety, can sabotage weight management efforts and lead to overeating.

- Strategy: Identify triggers for emotional eating and develop alternative coping strategies, such as practicing mindfulness, engaging in relaxation techniques, seeking support from friends or a therapist, or engaging in enjoyable activities that don't involve food.

3. Social and Environmental Influences:

- Challenge: Social situations, peer pressure, cultural norms, and environmental factors can influence eating behaviors and make it challenging to maintain healthy habits.

- Strategy: Plan ahead for social gatherings and choose healthier options when dining out. Surround yourself with supportive friends and family members who encourage healthy behaviors. Make changes to your home environment, such as keeping healthy snacks readily available and minimizing exposure to tempting foods.

4. Lack of Time and Convenience:

- Challenge: Busy schedules, work demands, and family responsibilities can make it difficult to prioritize healthy eating and physical activity.

- Strategy: Plan and prepare meals in advance, batch cook healthy recipes, and use time-saving cooking techniques such as slow cooking or meal prepping. Incorporate short bouts of physical activity into your daily routine, such as taking the stairs, walking during breaks, or doing quick home workouts.

5. Food Cravings and Temptations:

- Challenge: Cravings for high-calorie, sugary, or processed foods can derail weight management efforts and lead to overeating.

- Strategy: Practice mindful eating by tuning into your body's hunger and fullness cues and choosing foods that satisfy you without overindulging. Allow yourself occasional treats in moderation and focus on incorporating a variety of nutritious foods into your diet to prevent feelings of deprivation.

6. Plateaus and Setbacks:
  - Challenge: Weight loss plateaus, setbacks, and fluctuations are common and can be discouraging for individuals trying to lose weight.
  - Strategy: Focus on non-scale victories such as improvements in energy levels, mood, sleep quality, and overall well-being. Reassess your goals and strategies, make adjustments as needed, and stay committed to your long-term health and wellness journey.

7. Lack of Motivation or Support:
  - Challenge: Lack of motivation, accountability, or support from friends, family, or healthcare professionals can hinder progress in weight management.
  - Strategy: Find sources of motivation that resonate with you, whether it's achieving specific health goals, improving self-confidence, or setting a positive example for loved ones. Seek support from a registered dietitian, nutritionist, personal trainer, or weight loss support group to help you stay motivated and accountable.

8. Negative Self-Talk and Self-Sabotage:
  - Challenge: Negative self-talk, self-doubt, and self-sabotaging behaviors can undermine confidence and hinder progress in weight management.
  - Strategy: Practice self-compassion, positive affirmations, and cognitive reframing techniques to challenge negative thoughts and beliefs about yourself and your abilities. Focus on progress rather than perfection, and celebrate your achievements along the way.

9. Lack of Knowledge or Resources:
  - Challenge: Limited knowledge about nutrition, exercise, and healthy lifestyle habits can make it challenging to make informed decisions and adopt sustainable behaviors.
  - Strategy: Educate yourself about nutrition, portion control, meal planning, and physical activity through reputable sources such as registered dietitians, trusted websites, and evidence-based resources. Seek guidance from healthcare professionals or wellness professionals who can provide personalized advice and support.

10. Medical and Hormonal Factors:

- Challenge: Underlying medical conditions, hormonal imbalances, medications, or genetic factors can affect metabolism, appetite regulation, and weight management.
- Strategy: Consult with a healthcare provider or registered dietitian to address any underlying medical issues or hormonal imbalances that may be impacting weight management. Work with a healthcare team to develop a comprehensive plan that addresses your individual needs and health concerns.

Building a Positive Body Image Through Nutrition

Building a positive body image through nutrition involves adopting a holistic approach that focuses on nourishing your body, honoring its unique needs, and cultivating a healthy relationship with food. Here are some strategies to promote a positive body image through nutrition:

1. Focus on Health, Not Weight:
- Shift your focus away from the number on the scale and instead prioritize overall health and well-being. Embrace a health-centered approach to nutrition that emphasizes nourishing your body with nutrient-dense foods, staying physically active, and practicing self-care.

2. Practice Intuitive Eating:
- Listen to your body's hunger and fullness cues, and honor its signals of hunger, satiety, and satisfaction. Eat when you're hungry and stop when you're comfortably full, without rigid rules or restrictions. Trust your body's wisdom to guide your food choices and eating behaviors.

3. Reject Diet Culture:
- Challenge societal norms and messages that promote unrealistic beauty standards, restrictive dieting, and body shaming. Reject diet culture's emphasis on thinness and external validation, and instead embrace body positivity, self-acceptance, and self-love at any size.

4. Focus on Nutrient-Rich Foods:

- Prioritize nutrient-dense foods that nourish your body and support overall health and vitality. Include a variety of fruits, vegetables, whole grains, lean proteins, and healthy fats in your diet to ensure you're getting essential nutrients and energy for optimal functioning.

5. Practice Gentle Nutrition:

- Approach nutrition with a gentle and compassionate mindset, free from guilt, shame, or judgment. Strive for balance, flexibility, and moderation in your food choices, allowing yourself to enjoy a wide range of foods without labeling them as "good" or "bad."

6. Celebrate Food Diversity:

- Embrace food diversity and cultural traditions by exploring new cuisines, flavors, and cooking techniques. Celebrate the pleasure and enjoyment of eating by savoring your meals, engaging your senses, and appreciating the rich cultural heritage of food.

7. Reject Food Moralizing:

- Avoid moralizing food choices or attaching moral value to specific foods. Recognize that all foods can fit into a balanced diet, and there's no such thing as "good" or "bad" foods. Allow yourself to enjoy your favorite treats in moderation without guilt or shame.

8. Practice Mindful Eating:

- Cultivate mindfulness during meals by slowing down, savoring each bite, and paying attention to the taste, texture, and aroma of your food. Tune into your body's hunger and fullness signals, and eat with intention and awareness rather than on autopilot.

9. Focus on Non-Weight Related Goals:

- Set health-related goals that are not focused solely on weight or appearance. Instead, focus on behaviors that promote well-being, such as improving energy levels, enhancing fitness, reducing stress, improving sleep quality, or cultivating positive body image and self-esteem.

10. Seek Support and Professional Guidance:

- Surround yourself with supportive friends, family members, or professionals who uplift and affirm your worth beyond appearance.

Seek support from a registered dietitian, therapist, or counselor who can help you develop a healthy relationship with food and body image.

Chapter 14
Nutrition and Mental Health

The Gut-Brain Connection

The gut-brain connection refers to the bidirectional communication between the gastrointestinal tract (the gut) and the brain, which plays a crucial role in regulating various physiological processes, including digestion, mood, and mental health. Here's an overview of the gut-brain connection and its implications for overall well-being:

1. Gut Microbiota:
   - The gut is home to trillions of microorganisms, including bacteria, viruses, fungi, and other microbes, collectively known as the gut microbiota. These microbes play a key role in digestion, nutrient metabolism, immune function, and the production of neurotransmitters.

2. Neurotransmitter Production:
   - The gut microbiota produce and interact with neurotransmitters, such as serotonin, dopamine, and gamma-aminobutyric acid (GABA), which are chemical messengers that regulate mood, behavior, and cognitive function. Serotonin, in particular, plays a crucial role in mood regulation and is sometimes referred to as the "feel-good" neurotransmitter.

3. Gut Hormones:
   - The gut produces various hormones, including ghrelin, leptin, and peptide YY, which regulate appetite, hunger, and satiety signals. These hormones influence food intake, energy balance, and body weight, and they can also affect mood and emotional well-being.

4. Immune Function:
   - The gut is closely linked to the immune system, with approximately 70-80% of the body's immune cells residing in the gastrointestinal tract. The gut microbiota play a crucial role in modulating immune function, inflammation, and the body's response to pathogens and foreign invaders.

5. Stress Response:
   - The gut-brain axis is involved in the body's response to stress, with bidirectional communication between the brain and the gut influencing

stress hormones, such as cortisol and adrenaline. Chronic stress can disrupt gut function, alter the composition of the gut microbiota, and contribute to gastrointestinal disorders, such as irritable bowel syndrome (IBS).

6. Mental Health Disorders:

- Dysfunction in the gut-brain axis has been implicated in various mental health disorders, including depression, anxiety, schizophrenia, and autism spectrum disorders. Changes in gut microbiota composition, inflammation, and neurotransmitter imbalances may contribute to the development or exacerbation of these conditions.

7. Dietary Factors:

- Diet plays a significant role in shaping the gut microbiota and modulating gut-brain communication. Consuming a diverse range of fiber-rich foods, fermented foods, and prebiotic and probiotic-containing foods can promote a healthy gut microbiota and support mental health.
- Conversely, diets high in processed foods, sugar, unhealthy fats, and artificial additives may disrupt gut microbiota balance, increase inflammation, and negatively impact mood and cognitive function.

8. Lifestyle Factors:

- In addition to diet, other lifestyle factors, such as sleep, exercise, stress management, and social connections, can influence the gut-brain axis and mental health outcomes. Prioritizing a healthy lifestyle that supports gut health can have positive effects on mood, cognition, and overall well-being.

9. Therapeutic Interventions:

- Therapeutic interventions targeting the gut-brain axis, such as probiotics, prebiotics, dietary supplements, and gut-directed therapies, are being investigated for their potential to improve mental health outcomes. Emerging research suggests that modulating gut microbiota composition and function may offer new avenues for the treatment of mental health disorders.

10. Holistic Approach:

- Taking a holistic approach to health that considers the interconnectedness of the gut, brain, and other body systems is essential for promoting optimal mental health and well-being. By nourishing the gut with a balanced diet, managing stress, prioritizing sleep, staying physically active, and fostering supportive social connections, individuals can support gut-brain communication and enhance mental health outcomes.

Foods That Support Mental Well-Being

Foods play a crucial role in supporting mental well-being by providing essential nutrients that support brain function, neurotransmitter production, and overall mood regulation. Here are some foods that are known to support mental health and promote emotional well-being:

1. Fatty Fish:
  - Fatty fish such as salmon, mackerel, trout, sardines, and herring are rich in omega-3 fatty acids, particularly EPA (eicosapentaenoic acid) and DHA (docosahexaenoic acid), which are essential for brain health and function. Omega-3 fatty acids have been linked to reduced risk of depression and may help improve mood and cognitive function.

2. Leafy Greens:
  - Leafy green vegetables such as spinach, kale, Swiss chard, and collard greens are rich in folate (vitamin B9), which plays a key role in neurotransmitter synthesis, including serotonin and dopamine. Adequate folate intake has been associated with a reduced risk of depression and improved mood.

3. Berries:
  - Berries such as blueberries, strawberries, raspberries, and blackberries are rich in antioxidants, particularly flavonoids, which have been linked to improved cognitive function, reduced inflammation, and enhanced mood. Consuming berries regularly may help protect against age-related cognitive decline and promote overall brain health.

4. Nuts and Seeds:

- Nuts and seeds, including almonds, walnuts, flaxseeds, chia seeds, and pumpkin seeds, are rich in healthy fats, protein, fiber, vitamins, and minerals. They provide essential nutrients such as magnesium, zinc, and vitamin E, which support brain health and may help reduce symptoms of anxiety and depression.

5. Whole Grains:
  - Whole grains such as oats, quinoa, brown rice, barley, and whole wheat are rich in complex carbohydrates, fiber, and B vitamins, including thiamine, riboflavin, niacin, and vitamin B6. These nutrients are involved in energy metabolism and neurotransmitter production, which are important for mood regulation and cognitive function.

6. Legumes:
  - Legumes such as beans, lentils, chickpeas, and peas are excellent sources of plant-based protein, fiber, and complex carbohydrates. They also provide nutrients such as folate, magnesium, and iron, which support brain health and may help improve mood and reduce symptoms of depression.

7. Yogurt and Fermented Foods:
  - Yogurt, kefir, kimchi, sauerkraut, and other fermented foods are rich in probiotics, beneficial bacteria that support gut health and may influence brain function and mood. Emerging research suggests that the gut-brain axis plays a key role in mental health, and consuming probiotic-rich foods may help support a healthy microbiome and improve mood.

8. Dark Chocolate:
  - Dark chocolate with a high cocoa content (70% or higher) is rich in flavonoids, particularly flavanols, which have antioxidant and anti-inflammatory properties. Consuming dark chocolate in moderation may help improve mood, reduce stress, and enhance cognitive function by increasing blood flow to the brain and promoting the release of feel-good neurotransmitters such as serotonin and endorphins.

9. Avocados:
  - Avocados are rich in monounsaturated fats, which support brain health and may help improve mood and cognitive function. They also

provide nutrients such as vitamin E, potassium, and folate, which are important for overall well-being.

10. Herbal Teas:
  - Herbal teas such as chamomile, peppermint, lemon balm, and green tea are known for their calming and relaxing properties. Drinking herbal teas can help reduce stress, promote relaxation, and support mental well-being.

Nutritional Strategies for Stress Management

Nutritional strategies play a significant role in managing stress and supporting mental health. Here are some effective strategies to consider:

1. Balanced Diet:
  - Consuming a balanced diet rich in nutrient-dense foods provides the essential vitamins, minerals, and antioxidants needed for optimal brain function and stress management. Focus on incorporating a variety of fruits, vegetables, whole grains, lean proteins, and healthy fats into your meals.

2. Complex Carbohydrates:
  - Complex carbohydrates, such as whole grains (oats, brown rice, quinoa) and starchy vegetables (sweet potatoes, squash), can help regulate blood sugar levels and promote the production of serotonin, a neurotransmitter that regulates mood and promotes relaxation.

3. Omega-3 Fatty Acids:
  - Omega-3 fatty acids found in fatty fish (salmon, mackerel, sardines), flaxseeds, chia seeds, and walnuts have anti-inflammatory properties and support brain health. Incorporating omega-3-rich foods into your diet may help reduce stress and improve mood.

4. Magnesium-Rich Foods:
  - Magnesium plays a crucial role in regulating stress response and promoting relaxation. Foods high in magnesium include leafy greens, nuts and seeds (almonds, pumpkin seeds), legumes, whole grains, and

dark chocolate. Consuming magnesium-rich foods can help alleviate stress and anxiety.

5. Vitamin C-Rich Foods:
   - Vitamin C is an antioxidant that helps combat oxidative stress and supports the immune system. Citrus fruits (oranges, lemons, grapefruits), berries (strawberries, blueberries), kiwi, bell peppers, and broccoli are excellent sources of vitamin C and can help reduce stress levels.

6. Probiotic-Rich Foods:
   - Probiotics are beneficial bacteria that support gut health and may influence mood and stress response. Incorporating probiotic-rich foods such as yogurt, kefir, sauerkraut, kimchi, and kombucha into your diet can help support a healthy gut microbiome and improve stress resilience.

7. Herbal Teas:
   - Certain herbal teas, such as chamomile, peppermint, lemon balm, and lavender, have calming and relaxing properties. Drinking herbal teas can help promote relaxation, reduce stress levels, and improve sleep quality.

8. Hydration:
   - Staying hydrated is essential for overall health and stress management. Dehydration can exacerbate stress and impair cognitive function. Aim to drink plenty of water throughout the day and limit caffeine and alcohol intake, as they can contribute to dehydration and increase stress levels.

9. Limit Caffeine and Alcohol:
   - While moderate consumption of caffeine and alcohol may have temporary mood-enhancing effects, excessive intake can disrupt sleep patterns, increase anxiety, and exacerbate stress. Limiting caffeine and alcohol intake, particularly in the evening, can help promote relaxation and improve sleep quality.

10. Mindful Eating:

- Practicing mindful eating involves paying attention to hunger and fullness cues, savoring each bite, and eating with awareness. Mindful eating can help reduce stress levels, improve digestion, and enhance the enjoyment of meals.

The Role of Nutrition in Sleep Quality

Nutrition plays a significant role in sleep quality, impacting both the quantity and the quality of sleep. Here's how nutrition influences sleep:

1. Regulation of Sleep-Wake Cycle:
  - Certain nutrients play a role in regulating the body's sleep-wake cycle, including the production of neurotransmitters such as serotonin and melatonin. Serotonin, which is synthesized from the amino acid tryptophan, helps regulate mood and promotes relaxation, while melatonin is known as the "sleep hormone" that signals the body to prepare for sleep.

2. Foods That Promote Sleep:
  - Certain foods contain nutrients that support the production of serotonin and melatonin, promoting better sleep quality. Examples include:
    - Tryptophan-Rich Foods: Turkey, chicken, fish, eggs, dairy products, nuts, seeds, tofu, and legumes are high in tryptophan, which can help increase serotonin levels and promote relaxation.
    - Carbohydrates: Complex carbohydrates such as whole grains (oats, brown rice, quinoa), starchy vegetables (sweet potatoes, squash), and fruits can aid in the absorption of tryptophan and facilitate the production of serotonin.
    - Magnesium-Rich Foods: Magnesium helps relax muscles and calm the nervous system, promoting relaxation and better sleep. Foods high in magnesium include leafy greens, nuts and seeds, legumes, whole grains, and dark chocolate.

3. Timing of Meals and Snacks:
  - The timing and composition of meals and snacks can impact sleep quality. Consuming large, heavy meals close to bedtime can disrupt digestion and lead to discomfort, making it harder to fall asleep. It's

recommended to avoid heavy meals, caffeine, and alcohol in the hours leading up to bedtime to promote better sleep quality.

4. Hydration:

- Proper hydration is essential for overall health and can also impact sleep quality. Dehydration can lead to discomfort and disrupt sleep, so it's important to stay adequately hydrated throughout the day. However, it's advisable to limit fluid intake in the evening to avoid disruptions to sleep due to frequent trips to the bathroom.

5. Avoidance of Stimulants:

- Stimulants such as caffeine, nicotine, and certain medications can interfere with sleep by stimulating the nervous system and disrupting the body's natural sleep-wake cycle. It's advisable to limit or avoid caffeine-containing beverages (coffee, tea, energy drinks) and other stimulants in the afternoon and evening to promote better sleep quality.

6. Balancing Blood Sugar Levels:

- Fluctuations in blood sugar levels can impact sleep quality and lead to disruptions in sleep patterns. Consuming a balanced diet that includes complex carbohydrates, lean proteins, and healthy fats can help stabilize blood sugar levels and promote more restful sleep.

7. Mindful Eating:

- Practicing mindful eating, which involves paying attention to hunger and fullness cues, savoring each bite, and eating with awareness, can promote better digestion and enhance sleep quality. Avoiding overeating and heavy, rich foods close to bedtime can help prevent discomfort and promote relaxation.

8. Individual Variations:

- It's important to recognize that individual nutritional needs and sensitivities vary, and what works well for one person may not be suitable for another. Experimenting with different foods, meal timings, and eating patterns can help identify what works best for promoting better sleep quality.

Addressing Emotional Eating Habits

Addressing emotional eating habits involves developing awareness of the triggers and patterns associated with emotional eating and implementing strategies to cultivate a healthier relationship with food. Here are some strategies to help address emotional eating habits:

1. Identify Triggers:
  - Recognize the emotions, situations, or triggers that lead to emotional eating, such as stress, boredom, loneliness, sadness, or anxiety. Keeping a food diary can help identify patterns and triggers associated with emotional eating.

2. Practice Mindfulness:
  - Develop mindfulness skills to become more aware of your thoughts, feelings, and bodily sensations without judgment. Mindfulness techniques, such as deep breathing, meditation, and mindful eating, can help you pause and respond more intentionally to emotions instead of reacting impulsively with food.

3. Find Healthy Coping Mechanisms:
  - Explore alternative coping mechanisms and activities to manage emotions and stress without turning to food. Engage in activities that bring you joy, relaxation, and fulfillment, such as exercise, hobbies, spending time with loved ones, journaling, or practicing self-care.

4. Distinguish Physical Hunger from Emotional Hunger:
  - Learn to differentiate between physical hunger, which arises from the body's physiological need for nourishment, and emotional hunger, which stems from emotional or psychological cues. Ask yourself if you're truly hungry or if you're seeking comfort, distraction, or relief from emotions.

5. Create a Supportive Environment:
  - Surround yourself with a supportive environment that encourages healthy eating habits and emotional well-being. Seek support from friends, family members, or a therapist who can provide encouragement, understanding, and guidance in navigating emotional eating challenges.

6. Build Resilience Skills:

- Develop resilience skills to cope with stress and navigate challenging emotions more effectively. Practice self-compassion, positive self-talk, and stress management techniques to build emotional resilience and reduce reliance on food as a coping mechanism.

7. Practice Intuitive Eating:

- Embrace intuitive eating principles by listening to your body's hunger and fullness cues, honoring your cravings without judgment, and making peace with food. Focus on nourishing your body with balanced meals and snacks that satisfy both physical and emotional hunger.

8. Plan Ahead for Emotional Triggers:

- Anticipate and plan ahead for situations or triggers that may lead to emotional eating. Develop strategies to cope with stressors and emotions proactively, such as creating a list of alternative activities, practicing relaxation techniques, or seeking support from a trusted friend or therapist.

9. Address Underlying Issues:

- Consider seeking professional help to address underlying emotional issues, trauma, or psychological factors that contribute to emotional eating habits. Therapy, counseling, or support groups can provide insights, tools, and strategies to address emotional eating patterns and promote healing.

10. Practice Self-Care:

- Prioritize self-care practices that nourish your physical, emotional, and mental well-being. Engage in activities that promote relaxation, self-compassion, and stress reduction, such as getting adequate sleep, exercising regularly, practicing mindfulness, and setting boundaries.

Chapter 15
Common Dietary Challenges and Solutions

Overcoming Sugar Addiction

Overcoming sugar addiction can be challenging but is achievable with commitment, awareness, and strategic approaches. Here are some steps to help overcome sugar addiction:

1. Understand Sugar Addiction:
- Educate yourself about the effects of sugar on the body and brain. Understand how sugar affects neurotransmitters, such as dopamine, and how excessive sugar consumption can lead to cravings, mood swings, and energy crashes.

2. Identify Triggers:
- Recognize the triggers that lead to sugar cravings and consumption. These triggers may include stress, boredom, emotional eating, social situations, or habitual patterns. Keeping a food diary can help identify patterns and triggers associated with sugar consumption.

3. Gradual Reduction:
- Rather than trying to eliminate sugar abruptly, gradually reduce your sugar intake over time. Start by cutting back on sugary beverages, desserts, and processed foods high in added sugars. Replace sugary snacks with healthier alternatives such as fruits, nuts, or Greek yogurt.

4. Read Labels:
- Learn to read food labels and identify hidden sources of sugar in packaged foods. Be mindful of ingredients such as high-fructose corn syrup, cane sugar, sucrose, dextrose, and other syrups and sweeteners. Choose whole foods and minimize consumption of processed foods and sugary snacks.

5. Opt for Whole Foods:
- Base your diet on whole, nutrient-dense foods such as fruits, vegetables, whole grains, lean proteins, and healthy fats. Whole foods provide essential nutrients, fiber, and antioxidants that support overall health and help regulate blood sugar levels, reducing cravings for sugary foods.

6. Balance Macronutrients:

- Include a balance of macronutrients (carbohydrates, protein, and fat) in your meals to promote satiety and stabilize blood sugar levels. Consuming meals that contain protein, healthy fats, and fiber-rich carbohydrates can help reduce cravings and prevent blood sugar spikes and crashes.

7. Stay Hydrated:
- Drink plenty of water throughout the day to stay hydrated and reduce cravings for sugary beverages. Sometimes thirst can be mistaken for hunger or cravings, so staying hydrated can help curb unnecessary sugar consumption.

8. Manage Stress:
- Find healthy ways to manage stress and emotional eating, as stress can trigger cravings for sugary foods. Practice relaxation techniques such as deep breathing, meditation, yoga, or mindfulness to reduce stress levels and promote emotional well-being.

9. Get Adequate Sleep:
- Prioritize getting adequate sleep, as sleep deprivation can disrupt hunger hormones and increase cravings for sugary and high-calorie foods. Aim for 7-9 hours of quality sleep per night to support overall health and reduce sugar cravings.

10. Seek Support:
- Enlist the support of friends, family members, or a healthcare professional to help you overcome sugar addiction. Joining a support group, working with a registered dietitian, or seeking counseling can provide encouragement, accountability, and guidance on making sustainable dietary changes.

11. Practice Moderation:
- Allow yourself to enjoy sweet treats occasionally in moderation, without guilt or deprivation. Practice mindful eating and savor small portions of your favorite desserts or treats without overindulging. Focus on overall dietary patterns and long-term health goals rather than strict rules or deprivation.

Managing Salt Intake for Heart Health

Managing salt intake is crucial for heart health as excessive sodium consumption can increase blood pressure and contribute to cardiovascular diseases. Here are some strategies to help manage salt intake for heart health:

1. Understand Recommended Limits:
   - Familiarize yourself with recommended sodium intake guidelines. The American Heart Association (AHA) recommends limiting sodium intake to no more than 2,300 milligrams (mg) per day, with an ideal limit of 1,500 mg per day for most adults, especially those with high blood pressure, kidney disease, or other cardiovascular risk factors.

2. Read Food Labels:
   - Pay attention to food labels and choose lower-sodium options when shopping for groceries. Opt for products labeled "low sodium," "reduced sodium," or "no added salt." Be mindful of hidden sources of sodium in processed and packaged foods such as soups, sauces, condiments, snacks, and canned goods.

3. Cook at Home:
   - Prepare meals at home using fresh, whole ingredients to have better control over salt content. Use herbs, spices, citrus juice, vinegar, and other flavor-enhancing ingredients to season foods instead of relying on salt. Experiment with different herbs and spices to add depth and flavor to your dishes without adding extra sodium.

4. Limit Processed Foods:
   - Minimize consumption of processed and packaged foods, which tend to be high in sodium. These include fast food, frozen meals, processed meats, canned soups, salty snacks, instant noodles, and pre-packaged sauces and seasonings. Choose whole, minimally processed foods whenever possible.

5. Rinse Canned Foods:
   - If using canned beans, vegetables, or other canned foods, rinse them thoroughly under running water to remove excess sodium. This

can help reduce sodium content by up to 40% or more. Look for low-sodium or no-salt-added varieties when purchasing canned foods.

6. Be Mindful When Dining Out:
  - When eating out at restaurants, ask for dishes to be prepared without added salt or with minimal salt. Request sauces, dressings, and condiments on the side so you can control how much you add. Choose dishes that are grilled, baked, steamed, or broiled rather than fried or heavily seasoned.

7. Use Salt Substitutes Wisely:
  - Consider using salt substitutes or alternatives such as potassium-based substitutes or herb blends that mimic the taste of salt without the sodium. However, use these substitutes sparingly and consult with a healthcare professional, especially if you have kidney disease or other medical conditions.

8. Increase Potassium-Rich Foods:
  - Increase your intake of potassium-rich foods, as potassium helps counteract the effects of sodium on blood pressure. Include foods such as bananas, oranges, potatoes, sweet potatoes, spinach, tomatoes, avocados, and yogurt in your diet.

9. Pay Attention to Serving Sizes:
  - Be mindful of portion sizes when consuming salty foods. Even small amounts of high-sodium foods can contribute significantly to your daily sodium intake. Pay attention to serving sizes listed on food labels and consider using smaller plates and bowls to control portion sizes.

10. Monitor Blood Pressure:
  - Regularly monitor your blood pressure and consult with a healthcare professional if you have concerns about hypertension or cardiovascular health. Managing sodium intake, along with other lifestyle modifications such as regular exercise, weight management, and stress reduction, can help lower blood pressure and reduce the risk of heart disease.

Strategies for Reducing Processed Food Consumption

Reducing processed food consumption is essential for improving overall health and well-being. Here are some strategies to help you minimize processed foods in your diet:

1. Focus on Whole Foods:
- Base your meals around whole, minimally processed foods such as fruits, vegetables, whole grains, lean proteins, and healthy fats. These foods are nutrient-dense and provide essential vitamins, minerals, fiber, and antioxidants that support overall health.

2. Read Food Labels:
- Pay attention to food labels and ingredient lists when shopping for groceries. Choose products with shorter ingredient lists and recognizable, whole food ingredients. Avoid products with added sugars, artificial additives, preservatives, hydrogenated oils, and highly processed ingredients.

3. Cook at Home:
- Prepare meals at home using fresh, whole ingredients whenever possible. Cooking from scratch allows you to have full control over the ingredients and cooking methods used in your meals. Experiment with simple recipes and cooking techniques to create flavorful and nutritious meals at home.

4. Meal Prep and Planning:
- Plan your meals and snacks ahead of time to avoid relying on processed convenience foods when hunger strikes. Set aside time each week for meal prep and batch cooking to have healthy options readily available. Prepare and portion out ingredients and meals in advance to streamline mealtime.

5. Choose Healthy Snacks:
- Opt for whole food snacks such as fresh fruits, vegetables, nuts, seeds, yogurt, hummus, and whole grain crackers instead of processed

snack foods. Keep healthy snacks readily available and easily accessible
to help curb cravings and prevent reaching for processed options.

6. Limit Sugary Beverages:
   - Reduce consumption of sugary beverages such as soda, fruit juices,
sports drinks, and sweetened teas and coffees. These beverages are
often high in added sugars and provide empty calories. Opt for water,
herbal teas, sparkling water, or infused water as healthier alternatives.

7. Be Selective with Packaged Foods:
   - Choose packaged foods wisely and opt for minimally processed
options when necessary. Look for products with recognizable
ingredients and minimal added sugars, sodium, and unhealthy fats.
Compare labels and choose products with the lowest amount of
additives and preservatives.

8. Be Mindful When Dining Out:
   - When eating out at restaurants or ordering takeout, make healthier
choices by selecting dishes made with whole, fresh ingredients. Look
for menu options that include fruits, vegetables, lean proteins, and
whole grains. Ask for dressings, sauces, and condiments on the side to
control portions and avoid hidden additives.

9. Gradually Reduce Processed Foods:
   - Gradually reduce your intake of processed foods over time to allow
your taste buds to adjust to healthier, whole food options. Start by
replacing one processed food item with a whole food alternative each
week and gradually increase the amount of whole foods in your diet.

10. Stay Informed and Educated:
   - Stay informed about the health risks associated with processed
foods and the benefits of consuming whole, nutrient-dense foods.
Educate yourself about food labeling, marketing tactics, and the
impact of processed foods on overall health to make informed dietary
choices.

Dealing with Food Allergies and Intolerances

Dealing with food allergies and intolerances requires careful management to ensure proper nutrition while avoiding triggering foods. Here are some strategies to help navigate food allergies and intolerances:

1. Identify Trigger Foods:
- Work with a healthcare professional, such as an allergist or dietitian, to identify specific foods that trigger allergic reactions or intolerances. Keep a food diary to track symptoms and identify patterns related to certain foods or ingredients.

2. Read Labels Thoroughly:
- Read food labels carefully to identify potential allergens or ingredients that may trigger allergic reactions or intolerances. Look for allergen warnings and avoid foods that contain or may have come into contact with the allergen.

3. Educate Yourself:
- Learn about common food allergens and intolerances, as well as hidden sources of allergens in processed foods. Be aware of cross-contamination risks in restaurants, shared kitchen spaces, and food manufacturing facilities.

4. Plan Balanced Meals:
- Plan balanced meals that meet your nutritional needs while avoiding trigger foods. Focus on incorporating a variety of nutrient-dense foods that are safe for you to consume. Experiment with alternative ingredients and recipes to ensure variety in your diet.

5. Substitution and Alternatives:
- Identify suitable substitutions and alternatives for trigger foods to maintain a balanced diet. For example, if you're allergic to dairy, opt for plant-based milk alternatives such as almond milk, soy milk, or coconut milk.

6. Communicate Effectively:
- Communicate your food allergies and intolerances clearly with family members, friends, caregivers, and food service providers.

Educate them about your dietary needs and the importance of avoiding cross-contamination when preparing or serving food.

7. Be Prepared When Dining Out:
   - When dining out, inform restaurant staff about your food allergies or intolerances and ask about ingredient substitutions or modifications to accommodate your dietary needs. Choose restaurants that offer allergy-friendly options or have allergen menus available.

8. Carry Emergency Medications:
   - Carry emergency medications such as epinephrine injectors (EpiPens) or antihistamines if you have severe food allergies that may lead to anaphylaxis. Ensure that you and your caregivers know how to use these medications in case of an emergency.

9. Practice Safe Food Handling:
   - Practice safe food handling practices at home to minimize the risk of cross-contamination. Use separate utensils, cutting boards, and kitchen equipment for preparing allergen-free meals. Clean and sanitize surfaces thoroughly to prevent contamination.

10. Seek Professional Guidance:
   - Consult with a registered dietitian or nutritionist who specializes in food allergies and intolerances for personalized guidance and support. They can help you create a safe and balanced meal plan, address nutritional deficiencies, and navigate complex dietary restrictions.

11. Stay Positive and Flexible:
   - Stay positive and flexible in managing food allergies and intolerances. Focus on finding joy in safe and delicious foods that nourish your body and support your overall health. Be open to trying new foods and recipes to maintain variety in your diet.

Navigating Special Diets: Gluten-Free, Vegan, etc

Navigating special diets, such as gluten-free or vegan, requires careful planning to ensure adequate nutrition while avoiding restricted foods. Here are some strategies to help navigate these special diets:

1. Educate Yourself:
- Learn about the principles and guidelines of the specific diet you're following, whether it's gluten-free, vegan, paleo, or another dietary approach. Understand which foods are allowed and which should be avoided to ensure compliance with the diet.

2. Plan Balanced Meals:
- Plan balanced meals that meet your nutritional needs while adhering to the restrictions of your chosen diet. Focus on incorporating a variety of nutrient-dense foods, including fruits, vegetables, whole grains, legumes, nuts, seeds, and plant-based proteins.

3. Include Protein Sources:
- Ensure you're getting an adequate intake of protein by including plant-based protein sources such as beans, lentils, tofu, tempeh, edamame, nuts, seeds, and quinoa in your meals. If following a vegan diet, consider incorporating fortified foods or supplements to meet your protein needs.

4. Opt for Whole Foods:
- Base your diet on whole, minimally processed foods to ensure you're getting a variety of nutrients and avoiding hidden sources of gluten or animal products. Choose whole grains, fruits, vegetables, and plant-based proteins over processed and packaged foods.

5. Read Labels Carefully:
- Read food labels carefully to identify potential sources of gluten, animal products, or other restricted ingredients. Look for gluten-free or vegan certification labels to ensure products meet your dietary requirements. Be aware of hidden sources of gluten or animal-derived ingredients in processed foods.

6. Experiment with Recipes:
- Explore new recipes and cooking techniques to make delicious and satisfying meals that align with your dietary preferences and restrictions. Get creative with plant-based ingredients, herbs, spices, and seasonings to add flavor and variety to your dishes.

7. Supplement Wisely:
  - Consider supplementing your diet with vitamins or minerals that may be lacking due to dietary restrictions. For example, individuals following a vegan diet may need to supplement with vitamin B12, vitamin D, omega-3 fatty acids, iron, or calcium to meet their nutritional needs.

8. Be Prepared When Dining Out:
  - When dining out, research restaurant menus in advance and communicate your dietary restrictions with restaurant staff. Ask about ingredient substitutions or modifications to accommodate your special diet. Choose restaurants that offer gluten-free or vegan options, or be prepared to customize your order.

9. Focus on Nutrient-Rich Foods:
  - Prioritize nutrient-rich foods that provide essential vitamins, minerals, and antioxidants to support overall health and well-being. Include a variety of colorful fruits, vegetables, whole grains, legumes, nuts, and seeds in your diet to ensure you're meeting your nutritional needs.

10. Seek Support and Resources:
  - Connect with online communities, support groups, or local organizations that focus on the specific diet you're following. Share tips, recipes, and experiences with others who have similar dietary restrictions. Consider working with a registered dietitian or nutritionist who specializes in your chosen diet for personalized guidance and support.

Chapter 16
Eating Out and Social Situations

Making Healthy Choices at Restaurants

Making healthy choices at restaurants can be challenging, but with mindful decision-making, it's possible to enjoy a nutritious meal while dining out. Here are some tips for making healthier choices when eating at restaurants:

1. Plan Ahead:
   - Check the restaurant's menu online before going out to eat. Look for healthier options such as grilled or roasted proteins, salads, vegetable-based dishes, and whole grain options. Planning ahead can help you make informed choices and avoid impulsive decisions.

2. Choose Wisely:
   - Opt for dishes that are steamed, grilled, baked, or broiled instead of fried or sautéed in heavy sauces. Look for menu items that are rich in vegetables, lean proteins, and whole grains. Avoid dishes that are described as fried, breaded, creamy, or smothered in sauces.

3. Control Portions:
   - Be mindful of portion sizes when ordering. Consider sharing a larger entrée with a friend or asking for a half portion if available. Opt for smaller appetizers or side dishes instead of large entrees, and avoid supersized or all-you-can-eat options.

4. Start with Soup or Salad:
   - Begin your meal with a broth-based soup or a side salad with vinaigrette dressing. These options can help fill you up with nutrient-rich vegetables and fiber, reducing the likelihood of overeating during the main course.

5. Customize Your Order:
   - Don't be afraid to customize your order to meet your dietary preferences and needs. Ask for dressings, sauces, and condiments on the side so you can control the amount added to your meal. Request substitutions or modifications to make dishes healthier, such as replacing fries with steamed vegetables or whole grains.

6. Watch for Hidden Calories:

- Be mindful of hidden sources of calories, such as butter, cheese, and creamy sauces. Ask about how dishes are prepared and choose options that are lower in added fats, sugars, and sodium. Avoid toppings like bacon, fried onions, and excessive cheese.

7. Be Mindful of Beverages:

- Choose water, unsweetened tea, or sparkling water instead of sugary beverages like soda, lemonade, or sweetened iced tea. If you prefer alcoholic beverages, opt for light beer, wine, or spirits mixed with soda water or a splash of juice.

8. Control Temptations:

- Limit your intake of bread baskets, appetizers, and desserts, which can add extra calories and derail your healthy eating goals. Consider skipping the bread or appetizers altogether, or sharing a dessert with others to satisfy your sweet tooth without overindulging.

9. Practice Portion Control:

- If you're faced with large portion sizes, consider dividing your meal in half and saving the rest for later. Ask for a to-go box when your meal is served, or split an entrée with a dining companion to avoid overeating.

10. Listen to Your Body:

- Pay attention to your hunger and fullness cues throughout the meal. Eat slowly and savor each bite, stopping when you feel satisfied rather than overly full. Remember that it's okay to leave food on your plate if you're no longer hungry.

Strategies for Healthy Eating at Social Events

Maintaining healthy eating habits at social events can be challenging, but with some planning and strategies, it's possible to make nutritious choices while still enjoying yourself. Here are some tips for healthy eating at social events:

1. Plan Ahead:

- If you know you'll be attending a social event with food, plan ahead by eating a balanced meal or snack beforehand. This can help prevent overeating or making unhealthy choices due to hunger.

2. Bring a Healthy Dish:
- Offer to bring a nutritious dish to share with others. This ensures that there will be at least one healthy option available and allows you to control the ingredients used.

3. Survey the Options:
- Before filling your plate, take a look at all the available food options. Choose items that are rich in nutrients such as fruits, vegetables, lean proteins, and whole grains. Avoid or limit foods that are high in added sugars, unhealthy fats, and refined carbohydrates.

4. Practice Portion Control:
- Be mindful of portion sizes and avoid overeating. Use smaller plates and utensils to help control portions, and listen to your body's hunger and fullness cues.

5. Fill Up on Fruits and Vegetables:
- Load up on fruits and vegetables, which are low in calories and packed with essential vitamins, minerals, and fiber. Choose raw or lightly cooked vegetables and fresh fruit as healthy snack options.

6. Choose Lean Proteins:
- Opt for lean protein sources such as grilled chicken, fish, tofu, or beans. Protein helps keep you feeling full and satisfied, and it's essential for muscle repair and growth.

7. Watch Your Beverages:
- Be mindful of your beverage choices, as sugary drinks and alcoholic beverages can contribute a significant amount of calories. Choose water, unsweetened tea, or sparkling water as healthier alternatives, and limit alcohol consumption.

8. Practice Mindful Eating:

- Slow down and savor each bite, paying attention to the flavors, textures, and sensations of the food. Eating mindfully can help you enjoy your food more fully and prevent overeating.

9. Be Selective with Treats:
  - If there are indulgent treats or desserts available, be selective about which ones you choose to indulge in. Allow yourself to enjoy a small portion of your favorite treat without feeling guilty, but be mindful of portion sizes.

10. Stay Active:
  - Incorporate physical activity into your day, whether it's going for a walk, playing outdoor games, or dancing with friends. Staying active can help balance out any extra calories consumed at social events and promote overall health and well-being.

11. Practice Moderation:
  - Remember that it's okay to indulge occasionally, but aim for moderation and balance in your overall eating patterns. Don't feel guilty about enjoying special treats or foods at social events, but strive to make healthy choices most of the time.

Handling Peer Pressure and Dietary Preferences

Handling peer pressure and staying true to your dietary preferences can be challenging in social situations, but it's essential for maintaining your health and well-being. Here are some strategies to help you navigate peer pressure and stick to your dietary preferences:

1. Be Confident in Your Choices:
  - Have confidence in your dietary preferences and the reasons behind them. Remind yourself why you've chosen to eat a certain way, whether it's for health, ethical, or personal reasons.

2. Communicate Clearly:
  - Communicate your dietary preferences to your friends, family, and peers in a clear and assertive manner. Explain your reasons for

following a particular diet and politely decline offers of food that don't align with your preferences.

3. Offer Alternatives:
- Offer to bring your own food or suggest alternative dining options that cater to your dietary preferences. Propose restaurants or dishes that offer suitable options for everyone, allowing you to enjoy the meal together without compromising your dietary choices.

4. Educate Others:
- Take the opportunity to educate others about your dietary preferences and the benefits of healthy eating. Share information about the foods you enjoy and how they contribute to your overall health and well-being.

5. Stay Firm but Flexible:
- Stay firm in your dietary preferences, but be flexible when necessary. Understand that not everyone may share your dietary choices, and be willing to compromise or make adjustments to accommodate different preferences within the group.

6. Focus on the Positive:
- Focus on the positive aspects of your dietary preferences, such as improved health, energy levels, and ethical considerations. Emphasize the delicious and nutritious foods you enjoy rather than feeling deprived of certain foods.

7. Find Supportive Allies:
- Surround yourself with supportive friends and peers who respect your dietary preferences and encourage you to stay true to them. Seek out like-minded individuals who share similar dietary beliefs and can offer encouragement and understanding.

8. Practice Assertiveness:
- Practice assertive communication techniques to assert your dietary preferences without being confrontational or defensive. Use "I" statements to express your needs and boundaries, and be open to having respectful discussions about food choices.

9. Have a Backup Plan:
   - Have a backup plan in place for social situations where your dietary preferences may not be accommodated. Bring snacks or a small meal with you to ensure you have something to eat if suitable options aren't available.

10. Stay True to Yourself:
   - Ultimately, stay true to yourself and your values when it comes to food choices. Remember that your health and well-being are the most important priorities, and don't feel pressured to compromise them to fit in with others' expectations.

Balancing Indulgences with Nutritional Goals

Balancing indulgences with nutritional goals is an essential aspect of maintaining a healthy and sustainable approach to eating, especially in social situations. Here are some strategies to help you strike that balance:

1. Practice Moderation:
   - Allow yourself to enjoy occasional indulgences while maintaining overall moderation in your diet. Rather than completely avoiding your favorite treats, aim to enjoy them in smaller portions and less frequently.

2. Plan Ahead:
   - If you know you'll be indulging in a special meal or treat at a social event, plan your meals and snacks for the rest of the day accordingly. Choose lighter, nutrient-rich options leading up to the indulgence to balance out your overall intake.

3. Prioritize Nutrient-Dense Foods:
   - Focus on filling your plate with nutrient-dense foods such as fruits, vegetables, lean proteins, whole grains, and healthy fats. These foods provide essential vitamins, minerals, and fiber to support your overall health and well-being.

4. Be Mindful of Portions:

- Pay attention to portion sizes when indulging in treats or high-calorie foods. Enjoy smaller portions to satisfy your cravings without overindulging. Use smaller plates and utensils to help control portion sizes and prevent mindless overeating.

5. Listen to Your Body:

- Tune into your body's hunger and fullness cues to guide your eating decisions. Eat slowly, savoring each bite, and stop when you feel satisfied rather than overly full. Avoid eating out of boredom, stress, or emotional triggers.

6. Balance Your Plate:

- Aim for balance and variety in your meals by including a mix of carbohydrates, protein, and healthy fats. Incorporate colorful fruits and vegetables, lean proteins, and whole grains to provide a well-rounded mix of nutrients.

7. Stay Hydrated:

- Drink plenty of water throughout the day to stay hydrated and help curb cravings for unhealthy foods. Sometimes, feelings of hunger can be mistaken for thirst, so staying hydrated can help you differentiate between the two.

8. Practice Flexibility:

- Be flexible with your eating patterns and allow yourself to enjoy special occasions without guilt. Remember that one indulgent meal or treat won't derail your progress, as long as it's balanced with healthier choices the majority of the time.

9. Plan for Physical Activity:

- Incorporate physical activity into your routine to help offset the extra calories consumed from indulgences. Plan for a workout before or after a special meal or event to help balance out your energy intake and expenditure.

10. Be Kind to Yourself:

- Practice self-compassion and kindness towards yourself, especially when it comes to food choices. Avoid feelings of guilt or shame associated with indulging in treats, and focus on enjoying the experience without judgment.

Creating a Healthy Relationship with Food in Social Settings

Creating a healthy relationship with food in social settings is essential for maintaining overall well-being and enjoying dining experiences without guilt or stress. Here are some strategies to help you foster a positive relationship with food in social situations:

1. Practice Mindful Eating:
 - Be present and mindful during meals, paying attention to the flavors, textures, and sensations of the food. Eat slowly, savoring each bite, and listen to your body's hunger and fullness cues to guide your eating decisions.

2. Focus on Enjoyment:
 - Shift your focus from strict rules or restrictions to the enjoyment of food and socializing with others. Allow yourself to indulge in occasional treats or special meals without feelings of guilt or deprivation.

3. Honor Your Preferences:
 - Respect your dietary preferences and needs while also being open to trying new foods and experiences. Choose foods that nourish your body and align with your values, but don't be afraid to enjoy foods purely for pleasure on occasion.

4. Embrace Variety:
 - Embrace variety in your food choices and appreciate the diverse flavors and cuisines available in social settings. Explore different foods, flavors, and cultural dishes, and celebrate the richness of culinary experiences with friends and loved ones.

5. Practice Moderation:
 - Practice moderation in your food choices, allowing yourself to enjoy a balanced and varied diet without extremes or restrictions. Aim for

balance over time, rather than perfection in every meal or social occasion.

6. Plan Ahead:
  - Plan ahead for social events by considering your dietary preferences and the available food options. If necessary, eat a balanced meal or snack beforehand to help you make healthier choices and avoid overeating.

7. Set Boundaries:
  - Set boundaries around food-related conversations and behaviors that may trigger negative feelings or stress. Politely decline comments or questions about your food choices, and focus on enjoying the company of others rather than fixating on food.

8. Practice Self-Compassion:
  - Be kind to yourself and practice self-compassion when it comes to food and eating. Release feelings of guilt or shame associated with food choices, and forgive yourself for any perceived "mistakes" or deviations from your usual eating patterns.

9. Cultivate Awareness:
  - Cultivate awareness of your emotional and psychological relationship with food, exploring any underlying beliefs or attitudes that may influence your eating behaviors. Seek support from a therapist or counselor if you struggle with disordered eating or body image concerns.

10. Seek Support:
  - Surround yourself with supportive friends, family, or peers who respect your dietary choices and encourage a healthy relationship with food. Connect with like-minded individuals who share similar values and beliefs about food and nutrition.

Chapter 17
Nutrition Education and Resources

Reliable Sources for Nutrition Information

Reliable sources for nutrition information are crucial for obtaining accurate and evidence-based guidance on healthy eating. Here are some trusted sources you can turn to for reliable nutrition information:

1. Registered Dietitians (RDs) and Nutritionists:
  - Registered Dietitians (RDs) and nutritionists are trained professionals with expertise in nutrition and dietetics. They can provide personalized nutrition advice based on your individual needs and goals. Look for professionals who are credentialed and licensed in your area.

2. Government Agencies:
  - Government agencies such as the United States Department of Agriculture (USDA) and the Centers for Disease Control and Prevention (CDC) offer reliable nutrition information and dietary guidelines based on scientific research. These agencies provide evidence-based recommendations for healthy eating and disease prevention.

3. Academic Institutions:
  - Universities and research institutions conduct studies and publish research on various aspects of nutrition and health. Websites affiliated with academic institutions, such as university health centers and nutrition departments, often provide reliable information based on scientific evidence.

4. Professional Organizations:
  - Professional organizations offer trustworthy resources and guidelines on nutrition and health. These organizations consist of experts in the field who stay up-to-date on the latest research and developments in nutrition.

5. Health Care Providers:
  - Your healthcare provider, such as your doctor or a registered dietitian, can offer personalized nutrition advice tailored to your specific health needs and medical conditions. They can help you develop a nutrition plan that supports your overall health and addresses any dietary concerns or challenges.

6. Nutrition Websites and Portals:
   - Several reputable websites and online portals provide evidence-based nutrition information and resources.

7. Peer-Reviewed Journals:
   - Peer-reviewed scientific journals publish research studies and articles on nutrition-related topics. While these sources may be more technical, they provide valuable insights into the latest advancements and findings in nutrition science.

8. Public Health Campaigns:
   - Public health campaigns and initiatives often provide educational materials and resources on nutrition and healthy eating. Examples include campaigns focused on reducing obesity, promoting healthy eating habits, and raising awareness about the importance of fruits and vegetables in the diet.

9. Nutrition Apps and Tools:
   - Nutrition apps and tools can help track your food intake, analyze nutrient content, and provide guidance on healthy food choices. Look for apps developed by reputable organizations or endorsed by registered dietitians.

10. Critical Evaluation:
   - When evaluating nutrition information from any source, it's essential to critically assess the credibility of the information and consider the qualifications of the authors or organizations. Look for information that is based on scientific research, supported by reputable sources, and free from bias or commercial interests.

The Role of Registered Dietitians and Nutritionists

Registered Dietitians (RDs) and Nutritionists play a crucial role in providing evidence-based nutrition education and guidance to individuals seeking to improve their eating habits and overall health. Here's an overview of their roles and contributions:

1. Expertise in Nutrition Science:
   - Registered Dietitians (RDs) and Nutritionists have extensive education and training in nutrition science, including biochemistry, physiology, and metabolism. They understand how different nutrients affect the body and can provide accurate, science-based information on food and nutrition.

2. Individualized Nutrition Counseling:
   - RDs and Nutritionists offer personalized nutrition counseling tailored to each individual's unique needs, goals, and dietary preferences. They assess factors such as medical history, lifestyle, cultural background, and food preferences to develop customized nutrition plans.

3. Dietary Assessment and Planning:
   - RDs and Nutritionists conduct comprehensive dietary assessments to evaluate an individual's current eating habits and nutritional status. Based on this assessment, they develop personalized nutrition plans that promote optimal health and address specific dietary concerns or health conditions.

4. Nutrition Education and Counseling:
   - RDs and Nutritionists provide education and counseling on various aspects of nutrition, including macronutrients, micronutrients, portion sizes, meal planning, and food label reading. They empower individuals with the knowledge and skills needed to make informed food choices and adopt healthier eating habits.

5. Disease Prevention and Management:
   - RDs and Nutritionists play a key role in preventing and managing chronic diseases through nutrition therapy. They work with individuals at risk for or diagnosed with conditions such as obesity, diabetes, heart disease, and gastrointestinal disorders to develop nutrition interventions that support optimal health outcomes.

6. Nutritional Support for Special Populations:
   - RDs and Nutritionists provide specialized nutritional support for various populations, including children, pregnant and lactating women, athletes, older adults, and individuals with specific dietary needs or

medical conditions. They address unique nutritional requirements and provide guidance on meeting nutrient needs at different life stages.

7. Collaborative Care:
 - RDs and Nutritionists collaborate with other healthcare professionals, including doctors, nurses, therapists, and allied health professionals, to deliver integrated and coordinated care. They work as part of multidisciplinary teams to address complex health issues and promote holistic approaches to wellness.

8. Advocacy and Public Health Promotion:
 - RDs and Nutritionists advocate for policies and initiatives that promote public health and improve access to nutritious food and nutrition education. They participate in community outreach programs, public health campaigns, and legislative efforts aimed at addressing nutrition-related disparities and promoting healthy eating habits.

9. Continuous Professional Development:
 - RDs and Nutritionists are committed to lifelong learning and professional development to stay up-to-date on the latest research, trends, and developments in nutrition science. They participate in continuing education programs, attend conferences, and pursue advanced certifications to enhance their knowledge and skills.

10. Ethical and Evidence-Based Practice:
 - RDs and Nutritionists adhere to professional codes of ethics and standards of practice, ensuring that their recommendations are evidence-based, unbiased, and in the best interests of their clients' health and well-being. They prioritize transparency, integrity, and professionalism in their interactions with clients and colleagues.

Nutrition Apps and Online Tools

Nutrition apps and online tools have become an essential part of many people's efforts to maintain a healthy lifestyle, manage dietary requirements, or achieve fitness goals. These digital solutions offer a variety of features designed to support users in monitoring their dietary intake, planning meals, tracking physical activity, and gaining access to a wealth of nutritional information and advice. Here are some generic types of nutrition apps and online tools you might find:

Meal Trackers

These apps allow users to log their daily food intake, providing insights into their nutritional habits. Users can track calories, macronutrients (proteins, fats, carbohydrates), and micronutrients (vitamins and minerals) to ensure they're meeting their dietary goals.

Calorie Counters

Focused primarily on weight management, calorie counters help users maintain, gain, or lose weight by tracking calorie intake versus expenditure. They often include databases of foods with their calorie values and can integrate with wearable devices to track physical activity.

Recipe and Meal Planning Tools

These online tools offer a plethora of recipes tailored to various dietary needs and preferences, such as vegetarian, vegan, low-carb, or gluten-free diets. They can automatically generate shopping lists and meal plans to simplify users' weekly food preparation.

Nutrition Education Platforms

Aimed at increasing nutritional knowledge, these platforms provide articles, videos, and other educational materials on topics like healthy eating habits, the benefits of different nutrients, and how to read food labels.

Food Diary Apps

Similar to meal trackers, food diary apps focus more on the qualitative aspects of eating, encouraging users to reflect on their meals, hunger levels, and feelings associated with eating. This can help identify patterns and triggers for unhealthy eating habits.

Fitness and Nutrition Integration Apps

These apps combine nutrition tracking with fitness monitoring, allowing users to see the full picture of their health and fitness routine. They track workouts, steps, sleep, and diet, providing a holistic approach to health.

Specialized Dietary Apps
Catering to specific dietary needs, these apps are designed for individuals with allergies, intolerances, or conditions like diabetes. They offer features like barcode scanning to check for allergens or track blood sugar levels.

Social and Community Support Apps
Focusing on the motivational aspect, some apps incorporate social features allowing users to connect with friends or join communities with similar health and fitness goals. These platforms can offer challenges, rewards, and support from peers.

When choosing a nutrition app or online tool, it's important to consider your specific goals, needs, and preferences. Some apps offer a broad range of features, while others specialize in particular areas. It's also beneficial to look for apps that base their information and recommendations on scientific evidence and offer customization to fit your individual lifestyle and dietary requirements.

Books and Educational Materials on Nutrition

When seeking to expand your knowledge on nutrition, a plethora of books and educational materials are available that cover a wide range of topics within this vast field. These resources can cater to various interests and needs, from beginners looking to understand the basics of nutrition to professionals and students desiring in-depth scientific insights. Here are some types of books and educational materials on nutrition:

Introductory Books on Nutrition
These books are designed for individuals new to the topic, providing foundational knowledge about the principles of nutrition, the importance of various nutrients, and how diet affects overall health. They often include guidelines for healthy eating and tips for making nutritious choices.

Cookbooks with a Nutritional Focus
Cookbooks that emphasize nutrition offer recipes designed to be healthy, delicious, and nutritious. They often cater to specific dietary

preferences or needs, such as low-carb, gluten-free, vegetarian, or vegan diets, and include information on the nutritional content of each recipe.

Academic Textbooks on Nutrition
Geared towards students and professionals, academic textbooks cover the science of nutrition in depth. Topics may include biochemistry, physiology, food science, and dietetics. These texts are often used in college and university courses and can serve as valuable references for professionals in the health and wellness fields.

Specialized Books on Diet and Health Conditions
Some books focus on the relationship between diet and specific health conditions, such as heart disease, diabetes, or digestive health issues. They provide dietary recommendations, meal planning advice, and the latest research findings on how nutrition can support disease management or prevention.

Nutritional Science and Research Journals
For those interested in the latest scientific research in the field of nutrition, academic journals publish peer-reviewed articles on a wide range of topics, from the effects of specific nutrients on health to the impact of dietary patterns on disease prevention.

Guides to Nutritional Supplements
These materials offer information on various dietary supplements, including vitamins, minerals, herbs, and other substances. They discuss the potential health benefits, evidence supporting their use, recommended dosages, and safety considerations.

Online Courses and Webinars
Many institutions and health organizations offer online courses and webinars on nutrition, ranging from introductory classes to specialized topics. These can provide interactive learning experiences and the opportunity to earn certificates or continuing education credits.

Nutritional Policy and Public Health Publications
Books and reports that examine nutritional policy and public health issues discuss the impact of diet on population health, strategies for improving food systems, and policies to promote healthy eating habits.

When choosing books and educational materials on nutrition, consider your specific interests, the credibility of the authors or publishers, and the relevance of the information to your health and dietary goals. Look for resources that are based on current scientific evidence and offer practical advice that can be applied to daily life. Whether you're looking to improve your own health, support others in making healthier choices, or pursue a career in the field of nutrition, there's a wealth of information available to guide you on your journey.

The Importance of Continuous Learning in Nutrition

Continuous learning in nutrition is essential for staying informed about the latest research findings, dietary guidelines, and nutrition trends. Here's why it's important:

1. Keeping Up with Evolving Science:
   - Nutrition science is constantly evolving, with new research studies and findings emerging regularly. Continuous learning allows individuals to stay updated on the latest scientific evidence regarding the relationship between diet and health. This ensures that dietary recommendations are based on the most current and reliable information available.

2. Adapting to Changing Guidelines:
   - Dietary guidelines and recommendations may change over time as new evidence emerges and scientific understanding evolves. Continuous learning enables individuals to adapt to these changes and adjust their dietary habits accordingly. Staying informed about updated guidelines helps ensure that dietary choices align with current best practices for promoting health and preventing disease.

3. Addressing Emerging Health Issues:
   - Continuous learning allows individuals to stay informed about emerging health issues related to nutrition and diet. For example, learning about the impact of dietary factors on conditions such as obesity, diabetes, heart disease, and cancer can help individuals take

proactive steps to improve their health and reduce their risk of developing these conditions.

4. Enhancing Nutritional Literacy:
   - Nutritional literacy refers to an individual's understanding of nutrition-related concepts, including macronutrients, micronutrients, dietary patterns, and food labels. Continuous learning helps improve nutritional literacy by providing individuals with the knowledge and skills needed to make informed food choices and adopt healthier eating habits.

5. Fostering Lifelong Health Habits:
   - Lifelong health habits are built on a foundation of continuous learning and self-improvement. By staying informed about nutrition and health, individuals can cultivate habits that support their long-term well-being and vitality. Continuous learning fosters a mindset of curiosity, exploration, and growth, empowering individuals to make positive choices for their health throughout their lives.

6. Empowering Informed Decision-Making:
   - Continuous learning empowers individuals to make informed decisions about their diet and lifestyle. By understanding the scientific evidence behind dietary recommendations and health claims, individuals can critically evaluate information from various sources and make choices that align with their health goals and values.

7. Supporting Professional Development:
   - For healthcare professionals, researchers, educators, and nutrition professionals, continuous learning is essential for professional development and maintaining competency in their field. Continuing education courses, seminars, workshops, and conferences provide opportunities to deepen knowledge, expand skills, and stay current with advances in nutrition science and practice.

8. Cultivating a Growth Mindset:
   - Continuous learning fosters a growth mindset, which is essential for personal and professional development. Embracing a mindset of lifelong learning encourages individuals to seek out new information,

challenge assumptions, and explore innovative approaches to nutrition and health.

Chapter 18
Global Perspectives on Nutrition

Addressing Food Insecurity and Malnutrition

Addressing food insecurity and malnutrition is a critical aspect of nutrition worldwide. Here's an overview of strategies and initiatives aimed at tackling these challenges:

1. Food Assistance Programs:
  - Governments, international organizations, and NGOs implement food assistance programs to provide food aid to vulnerable populations, including those affected by poverty, conflict, natural disasters, and economic instability. These programs may include food distribution, cash transfers, food vouchers, and nutrition education to ensure access to adequate and nutritious food.

2. Agricultural Development:
  - Investing in agricultural development and food production can help increase food availability and improve access to nutritious foods. Supporting smallholder farmers, promoting sustainable agriculture practices, enhancing crop diversity, and strengthening food systems contribute to food security and nutrition outcomes, particularly in low-income and rural communities.

3. Nutrition Education and Behavior Change:
  - Nutrition education programs empower individuals and communities to make healthier food choices and adopt nutritionally balanced diets. These programs provide information on topics such as dietary diversity, breastfeeding, micronutrient supplementation, hygiene, and food safety. By promoting behavior change and improving nutritional literacy, they help prevent malnutrition and promote optimal health.

4. Micronutrient Supplementation:
  - Micronutrient supplementation programs target populations at risk of micronutrient deficiencies, such as vitamin A, iron, iodine, and zinc. These interventions provide essential nutrients through supplements, fortified foods, or biofortified crops to address specific nutrient gaps and prevent nutritional deficiencies, especially among women, children, and pregnant women.

5. School Feeding Programs:

- School feeding programs provide nutritious meals or snacks to school-age children to improve their nutritional status, health, and educational outcomes. These programs often target children from low-income families who may not have access to adequate food at home. In addition to addressing hunger, school feeding programs promote attendance, concentration, and academic performance.

6. Nutrition-Sensitive Interventions:

- Nutrition-sensitive interventions integrate nutrition goals into broader development initiatives, such as health care, education, water, sanitation, and hygiene (WASH), social protection, and women's empowerment programs. These multisectoral approaches address the underlying determinants of malnutrition, including poverty, inequality, inadequate healthcare, and lack of access to clean water and sanitation.

7. Community-Based Approaches:

- Community-based approaches engage local communities in identifying, prioritizing, and implementing solutions to food insecurity and malnutrition. These approaches leverage community resources, knowledge, and networks to promote sustainable food production, nutrition education, maternal and child health services, and support for breastfeeding and complementary feeding practices.

8. Policy and Advocacy:

- Advocacy efforts aim to raise awareness, mobilize political commitment, and advocate for policy changes to address the root causes of food insecurity and malnutrition. These efforts may include advocating for increased investment in nutrition, strengthening food and agriculture policies, promoting social protection measures, and addressing inequities in food access and distribution.

9. Global Partnerships and Collaboration:

- Collaboration among governments, international organizations, civil society, academia, and the private sector is essential for addressing food insecurity and malnutrition on a global scale. Through partnerships and coordination, stakeholders can leverage resources, expertise, and innovation to develop comprehensive, sustainable solutions that improve nutrition outcomes for all.

10. Sustainable Development Goals (SDGs):
 - The United Nations' Sustainable Development Goals (SDGs),
particularly Goal 2 (Zero Hunger) and Goal 3 (Good Health and Well-
being), provide a framework for addressing food insecurity and
malnutrition at the global level. Achieving these goals requires
collective action, investment, and commitment to ensuring that
everyone has access to safe, nutritious, and affordable food.

Cultural Influences on Dietary Habits

Cultural influences play a significant role in shaping dietary habits and
food choices around the world. Here's how cultural factors impact
nutrition:

1. Traditional Food Practices:
 - Cultural traditions and customs often dictate the types of foods
consumed, meal preparation methods, and eating rituals within a
community or society. Traditional food practices may be influenced by
factors such as geographic location, climate, historical heritage,
religious beliefs, and agricultural practices.

2. Culinary Heritage:
 - Culinary heritage reflects the unique food traditions, recipes, and
cooking techniques passed down through generations within a cultural
group or region. Traditional dishes and cooking methods are cherished
as a source of identity, pride, and cultural heritage, shaping dietary
preferences and culinary preferences.

3. Food Taboos and Restrictions:
 - Many cultures have specific food taboos, restrictions, or dietary
guidelines based on religious, cultural, or spiritual beliefs. These
taboos may dictate which foods are considered permissible or
forbidden, how foods are prepared and consumed, and the symbolism
associated with certain foods.

4. Festivals and Celebrations:

- Festivals, holidays, and special occasions often revolve around food and communal meals, serving as opportunities for families and communities to come together, celebrate cultural traditions, and share traditional dishes. Festive foods are often rich in symbolism and significance, reinforcing cultural identity and social cohesion.

5. Family and Social Dynamics:

- Family and social dynamics influence food choices, eating behaviors, and meal patterns within a cultural context. Cultural norms regarding mealtime etiquette, portion sizes, sharing food, and hospitality shape social interactions and relationships around food.

6. Migration and Acculturation:

- Migration and acculturation can lead to changes in dietary habits as individuals and communities adapt to new cultural environments. Acculturation may involve incorporating foods from the host culture, modifying traditional recipes to suit local ingredients, or maintaining culinary traditions as a way to preserve cultural identity.

7. Globalization and Food Choices:

- Globalization has led to increased cultural exchange, culinary diversity, and access to a wide range of foods from around the world. As people become exposed to different cuisines and culinary traditions, their food preferences and dietary habits may evolve, reflecting a blend of cultural influences.

8. Food Marketing and Media:

- Food marketing, advertising, and media play a significant role in shaping food preferences and consumption patterns, particularly among younger generations. Cultural representations of food in the media, such as television, movies, and social media, can influence perceptions of food quality, desirability, and cultural value.

9. Environmental and Economic Factors:

- Environmental and economic factors, such as availability of local foods, access to resources, and socioeconomic status, influence food choices and dietary patterns within a cultural context. Limited access to nutritious foods, economic constraints, and environmental factors may contribute to dietary disparities and health inequities.

10. Cultural Competency in Nutrition Education:
 - Recognizing and understanding cultural influences on dietary habits
is essential for providing culturally sensitive and appropriate nutrition
education and counseling. Cultural competency in nutrition practice
involves respecting cultural diversity, tailoring interventions to meet
individual and community needs, and incorporating cultural beliefs and
preferences into dietary recommendations.

Sustainable Nutrition Practices

Sustainable nutrition practices aim to promote food security, protect
the environment, and support human health both now and in the
future. Here are key aspects of sustainable nutrition practices:

1. Balanced and Diverse Diets:
 - Sustainable diets emphasize the consumption of a variety of foods
from different food groups, including fruits, vegetables, whole grains,
legumes, nuts, seeds, lean proteins, and healthy fats. By diversifying
food sources, individuals can ensure adequate nutrient intake while
reducing reliance on resource-intensive foods.

2. Plant-Based Eating Patterns:
 - Plant-based eating patterns, such as vegetarian and vegan diets,
promote the consumption of plant-derived foods while minimizing or
eliminating animal products. Plant-based diets have lower
environmental footprints compared to animal-based diets, as they
require fewer natural resources, produce fewer greenhouse gas
emissions, and have less impact on land and water resources.

3. Locally Sourced and Seasonal Foods:
 - Choosing locally sourced and seasonal foods reduces the
environmental impact associated with long-distance transportation,
refrigeration, and storage of food. Buying locally grown produce and
supporting local farmers and food producers also strengthens local
economies and fosters community resilience.

4. Sustainable Food Production:

- Sustainable food production practices focus on minimizing environmental degradation, conserving natural resources, and promoting biodiversity. These practices may include organic farming methods, agroecology, permaculture, crop rotation, integrated pest management, and water conservation techniques.

5. Minimizing Food Waste:

- Minimizing food waste is essential for reducing the environmental footprint of food production and consumption. Strategies to reduce food waste include meal planning, proper storage, portion control, using leftovers creatively, composting organic waste, and supporting food recovery and redistribution initiatives.

6. Ethical Practices:

- Supporting ethical practices ensures that food producers receive fair wages, work in safe conditions, and adhere to sustainable agricultural practices. Choosing products with third-party certifications promotes social equity and environmental stewardship in the food supply chain.

7. Sustainable Seafood Choices:

- Making sustainable seafood choices helps protect marine ecosystems and fish populations from overfishing and habitat destruction. Consumers can look for eco-labels to identify responsibly sourced seafood options.

8. Reducing Animal Product Consumption:

- Limiting consumption of animal products, particularly red meat and processed meats, can reduce greenhouse gas emissions, water usage, and land degradation associated with livestock production. Choosing plant-based protein sources, such as legumes, tofu, tempeh, and nuts, can help lower environmental impact while promoting health.

9. Advocacy and Policy Change:

- Advocating for policies that support sustainable food systems, promote healthy eating habits, and address food insecurity is essential for creating lasting change at the societal level. Policy interventions may include subsidies for sustainable agriculture, incentives for local food production, regulations on food labeling and advertising, and initiatives to reduce food waste.

10. Education and Awareness:
 - Educating consumers, food producers, policymakers, and other stakeholders about the importance of sustainable nutrition practices fosters greater awareness and understanding of the links between food, health, and the environment. By raising awareness and promoting behavior change, individuals can contribute to building more sustainable food systems and creating a healthier, more resilient future for all.

Global Nutrition Initiatives and Challenges

Global nutrition initiatives aim to address malnutrition, improve food security, and promote healthy eating habits worldwide. However, several challenges persist in achieving these goals. Here's an overview:

Global Nutrition Initiatives:

1. School Feeding Programs: These programs provide meals to children in schools, ensuring they receive essential nutrients that support their growth and cognitive development. This not only helps in fighting child malnutrition but also increases school attendance and performance.

2. Maternal and Infant Nutrition: Initiatives focusing on the first 1,000 days of life, from pregnancy to a child's second year, emphasize the importance of adequate nutrition for pregnant and breastfeeding women, as well as infants. Such initiatives might provide supplements, education on breastfeeding, and access to nutritious foods.

3. Fortification of Foods: Adding essential vitamins and minerals to commonly consumed foods, such as flour, rice, or cooking oil, can address micronutrient deficiencies in large populations. This is a cost-effective way to improve public health outcomes.

4. Agricultural Development Programs: By supporting sustainable agricultural practices, these programs aim to increase food security, improve access to nutritious foods, and boost the incomes of smallholder farmers. This might include training on crop diversification, pest management, and climate-resilient farming techniques.

5. Nutrition Education and Behavior Change: Initiatives that focus on educating communities about nutrition can help change dietary behaviors. These might involve campaigns to promote the consumption of fruits and vegetables, cooking demonstrations, or nutrition classes in schools.

6. Food Aid and Emergency Nutrition Response: In crisis situations, such as natural disasters or conflicts, initiatives might provide food aid to affected populations. This can include the distribution of food parcels, ready-to-use therapeutic foods for treating acute malnutrition, and setting up feeding centers.

7. Public-Private Partnerships (PPPs): Collaborations between governments and the private sector can leverage resources and expertise to address malnutrition. This might involve developing nutritious products, improving food supply chains, or investing in food processing to preserve the nutritional quality of foods.

8. Global Health Initiatives: Some programs are dedicated to specific health outcomes related to nutrition, such as combating vitamin A deficiency, anemia, or obesity. These initiatives might involve targeted supplementation, public health campaigns, and policy-making to promote healthier food environments.

Challenges:

1. Persistent Malnutrition:
   - Despite efforts to address malnutrition, millions of people worldwide still suffer from undernutrition, micronutrient deficiencies, and overweight/obesity-related health problems. Malnutrition remains a complex and persistent challenge, particularly in low-income countries and marginalized populations.

2. Food Insecurity and Poverty:

- Food insecurity and poverty are major drivers of malnutrition, limiting access to nutritious foods, clean water, and essential health services for millions of people worldwide. Addressing the root causes of food insecurity requires comprehensive strategies that tackle poverty, inequality, and social disparities.

3. Nutrition Transition and Dietary Shifts:

- Rapid urbanization, globalization, and changing dietary patterns are contributing to shifts in food consumption towards energy-dense, processed foods high in sugar, salt, and unhealthy fats. These dietary transitions increase the risk of diet-related non-communicable diseases (NCDs), such as obesity, diabetes, and cardiovascular diseases, posing significant public health challenges.

4. Climate Change and Environmental Degradation:

- Climate change, environmental degradation, and natural disasters threaten food production, disrupt food systems, and exacerbate food insecurity and malnutrition. Extreme weather events, droughts, floods, and soil degradation can undermine agricultural productivity, compromise food safety, and disrupt supply chains, particularly in vulnerable regions.

5. Conflict and Humanitarian Crises:

- Conflict, displacement, and humanitarian crises exacerbate food insecurity, malnutrition, and health disparities, particularly among refugees, internally displaced persons (IDPs), and marginalized communities. Access to food, clean water, and essential health services is often compromised in conflict-affected areas, leading to acute malnutrition and humanitarian emergencies.

6. Inequities in Nutrition Access and Coverage:

- Inequities in nutrition access, coverage, and quality of care persist within and between countries, with marginalized populations, women, children, and rural communities facing disproportionate barriers to accessing nutritious foods, healthcare services, and nutrition interventions. Addressing these inequities requires targeted strategies that prioritize vulnerable groups and ensure universal access to essential nutrition services.

Building Healthy Diets in Diverse Societies

Building healthy diets in diverse societies requires consideration of cultural, socioeconomic, environmental, and individual factors. Here are key strategies for promoting healthy eating habits in diverse populations:

1. Cultural Sensitivity:
   - Recognize and respect cultural diversity in dietary preferences, food traditions, and eating habits. Tailor nutrition education and dietary recommendations to reflect cultural norms, beliefs, and preferences, emphasizing the importance of traditional foods and culinary practices in promoting health.

2. Dietary Diversity:
   - Encourage consumption of a variety of foods from different food groups to ensure a balanced and nutrient-rich diet. Promote dietary diversity by including fruits, vegetables, whole grains, legumes, nuts, seeds, lean proteins, and healthy fats in meals and snacks.

3. Traditional Foods and Culinary Heritage:
   - Emphasize the nutritional value and health benefits of traditional foods and culinary heritage. Highlight the importance of incorporating locally grown, seasonal, and culturally significant foods into daily meals, while preserving traditional cooking techniques and recipes.

4. Access to Nutritious Foods:
   - Address barriers to accessing nutritious foods, such as limited availability, affordability, and food insecurity. Promote equitable access to healthy foods by supporting local food systems, farmers' markets, community gardens, and initiatives that increase access to fresh, affordable produce in underserved areas.

5. Nutrition Education and Literacy:
   - Provide culturally appropriate nutrition education and resources that empower individuals and communities to make informed food choices and adopt healthy eating habits. Promote nutrition literacy, cooking skills, meal planning, and label reading to enhance understanding of nutrition and dietary guidelines.

6. Social and Environmental Factors:
   - Consider social and environmental determinants of health that influence dietary behaviors, such as income, education, food environments, marketing practices, and food policies. Advocate for policies and interventions that create supportive environments for healthy eating, such as nutrition labeling, school nutrition programs, and regulations on unhealthy food marketing.

7. Community Engagement and Participation:
   - Engage communities in designing and implementing nutrition interventions that address local needs, preferences, and priorities. Foster community ownership, participation, and collaboration in promoting healthy eating behaviors through grassroots initiatives, social networks, and community-based programs.

8. Health Equity and Social Justice:
   - Address disparities in access to healthy food and healthcare services by promoting health equity and social justice. Advocate for policies and programs that address underlying social determinants of health, such as poverty, inequality, discrimination, and structural barriers to health equity.

9. Sustainable Food Systems:
   - Promote sustainable food production and consumption practices that support human health, environmental sustainability, and social equity. Encourage consumption of plant-based foods, reduce food waste, support regenerative agriculture, and advocate for policies that promote sustainable food systems at local, national, and global levels.

10. Lifelong Healthy Eating Habits:
   - Foster lifelong healthy eating habits by promoting positive attitudes towards food, cooking, and eating, starting from early childhood through adulthood and into older age. Emphasize the importance of role modeling, family meals, school nutrition programs, workplace wellness initiatives, and community-based interventions in shaping dietary behaviors and preventing diet-related diseases.

Chapter 19
Ethical and Environmental Considerations in Nutrition

Sustainable Food Choices

Sustainable food choices are essential for promoting environmental conservation, protecting natural resources, and supporting ethical and equitable food systems. Here are key principles and practices for making sustainable food choices:

1. Plant-Based Diet:
- Incorporate more plant-based foods into your diet, such as fruits, vegetables, legumes, whole grains, nuts, and seeds. Plant-based diets have a lower environmental footprint compared to diets high in animal products, as they require fewer resources, produce fewer greenhouse gas emissions, and have less impact on land and water resources.

2. Locally Sourced Foods:
- Choose locally sourced and seasonal foods whenever possible to reduce the environmental impact associated with long-distance transportation, refrigeration, and storage of food. Buying from local farmers and producers supports regional economies, promotes food sovereignty, and strengthens community resilience.

3. Organic and Sustainable Agriculture:
- Support organic and sustainable farming practices that prioritize soil health, biodiversity conservation, and natural resource stewardship. Look for organic certifications and labels that indicate environmentally friendly farming methods, such as organic, regenerative agriculture, and agroecology.

4. Fair Trade and Ethical Certifications:
- Purchase foods with fair trade and ethical certifications to support fair wages, safe working conditions, and environmentally sustainable practices in the global food supply chain. Fair trade certifications ensure that producers receive fair compensation for their labor and adhere to social and environmental standards.

5. Sustainable Seafood Choices:
- Choose sustainably sourced seafood options that are harvested or farmed using responsible fishing and aquaculture practices. Look for

eco-labels to identify seafood products that meet environmental sustainability criteria.

6. Minimize Food Waste:

- Minimize food waste by planning meals, storing food properly, using leftovers creatively, and composting organic waste. Food waste contributes to greenhouse gas emissions, wastes valuable resources, and exacerbates environmental degradation. By reducing food waste, you can conserve resources and save money.

7. Seasonal Eating:

- Eat seasonally and enjoy foods that are in season and locally available. Seasonal eating not only supports local agriculture and reduces the carbon footprint associated with food transportation but also allows you to enjoy fresh, flavorful produce at its peak ripeness.

8. Reduce Packaging Waste:

- Choose foods with minimal packaging or opt for eco-friendly packaging options, such as bulk bins, reusable containers, and compostable packaging materials. Minimizing packaging waste helps reduce plastic pollution, conserve resources, and protect ecosystems.

9. Support Sustainable Food Systems:

- Advocate for policies and initiatives that promote sustainable food systems, such as organic farming subsidies, agroecological research, local food procurement policies, and regulations on food labeling and advertising. Support organizations and movements that advocate for sustainable agriculture, food justice, and environmental conservation.

10. Consumer Education and Awareness:

- Stay informed about sustainability issues related to food production, agriculture, and food systems. Educate yourself and others about the environmental impact of food choices, the importance of biodiversity conservation, and the benefits of sustainable farming practices. By raising awareness and promoting consumer behavior change, individuals can contribute to building a more sustainable food system for future generations.

The Impact of Food Production on the Environment

Food production has significant environmental impacts across various stages of the food supply chain, from agricultural practices to food processing, distribution, consumption, and waste management. Here are some key ways in which food production affects the environment:

1. Land Use and Deforestation:
   - Agriculture is a major driver of deforestation, habitat loss, and land degradation, particularly in tropical regions where forests are cleared for crop cultivation, livestock grazing, and agribusiness expansion. Deforestation contributes to biodiversity loss, soil erosion, and disruption of ecosystems, with implications for wildlife habitat, carbon sequestration, and climate regulation.

2. Greenhouse Gas Emissions:
   - Agriculture is a significant source of greenhouse gas (GHG) emissions, primarily from livestock production, soil management practices, fertilizer use, and rice cultivation. Livestock farming, especially cattle, emits methane, a potent greenhouse gas, while fertilizer application releases nitrous oxide, another potent greenhouse gas. Deforestation for agriculture also releases carbon dioxide (CO_2) stored in forests.

3. Water Use and Pollution:
   - Agriculture accounts for a substantial portion of global water use, both for irrigation and livestock watering. Excessive water extraction for agriculture can deplete freshwater resources, reduce water availability for other uses, and contribute to water scarcity in arid and semi-arid regions. Agricultural runoff containing fertilizers, pesticides, and animal waste can also pollute water bodies, leading to eutrophication, algal blooms, and degradation of aquatic ecosystems.

4. Soil Degradation and Loss of Fertility:
   - Unsustainable agricultural practices, such as intensive tillage, monocropping, and excessive use of chemical inputs, can degrade soil health, reduce soil fertility, and increase erosion rates. Soil erosion leads to loss of topsoil, nutrient depletion, and decreased agricultural

productivity, posing long-term challenges for food security and sustainable land management.

5. Biodiversity Loss and Habitat Destruction:
   - Agriculture contributes to habitat destruction, fragmentation, and loss of biodiversity through conversion of natural ecosystems into cropland, pastureland, and agricultural landscapes. Loss of biodiversity undermines ecosystem resilience, disrupts ecological processes, and increases vulnerability to pests, diseases, and climate change impacts.

6. Energy Consumption and Resource Use:
   - Food production, processing, and distribution require significant energy inputs, including fossil fuels for machinery, transportation, and refrigeration. Energy-intensive agricultural practices, such as irrigation pumping and mechanized farming, contribute to greenhouse gas emissions and resource depletion. Sustainable farming practices, such as agroecology and organic farming, can reduce energy use and reliance on fossil fuels.

7. Food Waste and Losses:
   - Food production systems contribute to food waste and losses at various stages of the supply chain, including harvesting, processing, storage, distribution, and consumption. Food waste not only represents a waste of resources, water, and energy invested in food production but also generates methane emissions when disposed of in landfills, exacerbating climate change.

8. Climate Change and Adaptation:
   - Climate change poses risks to food production systems through altered weather patterns, temperature extremes, water scarcity, and increased frequency of extreme events, such as droughts, floods, and heatwaves. Sustainable agricultural practices, such as climate-smart agriculture, agroforestry, and conservation agriculture, can help build resilience to climate change and mitigate its impacts on food security and livelihoods.

9. Pesticide and Chemical Pollution:
   - Intensive use of synthetic pesticides, herbicides, and fertilizers in conventional agriculture can lead to soil contamination, water

pollution, and adverse effects on human health and ecosystems. Organic farming and agroecological approaches promote reduced pesticide use, integrated pest management, and natural soil fertility enhancement methods, reducing environmental pollution and ecological risks.

10. Solutions and Sustainable Practices:
 - Transitioning to more sustainable food production practices, such as agroecology, organic farming, regenerative agriculture, and agroforestry, can help mitigate environmental impacts, conserve natural resources, and promote biodiversity conservation. Supporting local and small-scale food producers, reducing food waste, promoting plant-based diets, and adopting circular economy principles in food systems are also key strategies for building more environmentally sustainable and resilient food systems.

Ethical Considerations in Food Industry Practices

Ethical considerations in the food industry encompass a range of principles and practices aimed at promoting fairness, transparency, social responsibility, and ethical treatment of workers, animals, and the environment. Here are some key ethical considerations in food industry practices:

1. Fair Labor Practices:
 - Ensuring fair wages, safe working conditions, and labor rights for agricultural workers, food producers, and food industry employees. Addressing issues such as labor exploitation, forced labor, child labor, and precarious employment in the food supply chain.

2. Animal Welfare:
 - Promoting humane treatment of animals in food production systems, including livestock farming, poultry production, and fisheries. Adopting animal welfare standards, such as access to clean water, proper nutrition, adequate space, and humane slaughter practices, to minimize suffering and improve animal well-being.

3. Sustainable Sourcing:

- Supporting ethical sourcing practices that prioritize environmental sustainability, biodiversity conservation, and social equity. Promoting fair trade, organic farming, sustainable seafood, and responsible sourcing of agricultural commodities to ensure ethical supply chains and minimize negative impacts on ecosystems and communities.

4. Food Safety and Quality:

- Upholding standards of food safety, hygiene, and quality assurance to protect consumer health and well-being. Implementing food safety regulations, quality control measures, and traceability systems to prevent contamination, adulteration, and foodborne illnesses throughout the food production and distribution process.

5. Transparency and Labeling:

- Providing transparent information to consumers about the origin, production methods, and ingredients of food products. Labeling products with clear and accurate information, including nutritional content, allergen warnings, ethical certifications, and sustainability labels, to enable informed food choices and promote transparency in the marketplace.

6. Corporate Social Responsibility:

- Practicing corporate social responsibility (CSR) by integrating ethical, social, and environmental considerations into business operations, supply chain management, and decision-making processes. Engaging in philanthropy, community engagement, sustainable business practices, and ethical marketing to contribute positively to society and address social and environmental challenges.

7. Food Justice and Equity:

- Advancing food justice and equity by addressing systemic inequalities, food insecurity, and disparities in access to healthy, affordable food. Supporting initiatives that promote food sovereignty, community empowerment, and equitable food access for marginalized and underserved populations, including low-income communities, rural areas, and food deserts.

8. Consumer Empowerment:

- Empowering consumers to make ethical food choices by providing education, information, and resources on ethical and sustainable food practices. Encouraging consumer activism, ethical consumerism, and demand for ethically produced, environmentally friendly, and socially responsible food products.

9. Accountability and Transparency:
  - Holding food companies, producers, and policymakers accountable for ethical lapses, environmental violations, and human rights abuses in the food industry. Advocating for greater transparency, accountability, and regulatory oversight to ensure ethical behavior, compliance with labor standards, and respect for human rights throughout the food supply chain.

10. Collaboration and Advocacy:
  - Collaborating with stakeholders across the food system, including governments, businesses, civil society organizations, and consumers, to promote ethical practices, sustainable food systems, and ethical considerations in food policy and governance. Engaging in advocacy, public awareness campaigns, and multi-stakeholder initiatives to drive positive change and advance ethical values in the food industry.

Supporting Local and Fair Trade Practices

Supporting local and fair trade practices in nutrition is not only beneficial for the environment but also promotes social justice and economic sustainability. Here's how you can do it:

1. Buying Locally Grown Foods:
  - Purchase fruits, vegetables, grains, and other food products grown or produced locally. Buying local reduces carbon emissions associated with transportation, supports local farmers and economies, and ensures fresher, seasonal produce.

2. Participating in Farmers' Markets:
  - Visit farmers' markets in your community to buy directly from local farmers and producers. Farmers' markets offer a wide variety of fresh, locally sourced foods, including fruits, vegetables, dairy products,

meats, and artisanal goods. By shopping at farmers' markets, you can support small-scale farmers and artisans while enjoying high-quality, sustainably produced foods.

3. Joining Community Supported Agriculture (CSA) Programs:
- Consider joining a Community Supported Agriculture (CSA) program, where you can purchase a share of a local farm's harvest in advance and receive regular deliveries of fresh, seasonal produce throughout the growing season. CSA programs provide a direct connection between consumers and farmers, support sustainable farming practices, and promote food sovereignty and community resilience.

4. Supporting Fair Trade Products:
- Choose fair trade-certified products, such as coffee, tea, chocolate, bananas, sugar, and spices, which adhere to social, environmental, and labor standards that promote fair wages, safe working conditions, and environmental sustainability in producer communities. Look for fair trade labels to ensure that your purchases support ethical trade practices and improve the livelihoods of small-scale farmers and workers in developing countries.

5. Patronizing Local Food Cooperatives:
- Shop at local food cooperatives or co-ops that prioritize local sourcing, fair trade, and sustainable practices. Food cooperatives are member-owned and operated grocery stores that emphasize community engagement, democratic decision-making, and ethical business practices. By supporting food cooperatives, you can contribute to a more equitable and sustainable food system while accessing high-quality, locally sourced foods.

6. Eating Seasonally and Regionally:
- Embrace seasonal and regional eating by choosing foods that are in season and locally available. Eating seasonally reduces the environmental impact of food production, supports local agriculture, and promotes biodiversity conservation. Enjoying foods that are grown or produced in your region also connects you to your local food system and fosters a sense of place and cultural identity.

7. Promoting Food Justice and Equity:

- Advocate for policies and initiatives that promote food justice, equity, and access to healthy, affordable food for all communities. Support initiatives that address food insecurity, promote food sovereignty, and empower marginalized and underserved populations, including low-income communities, people of color, and indigenous communities, to access fresh, nutritious foods and participate in local food systems.

8. Educating Yourself and Others:
- Learn more about the benefits of supporting local and share the knowledge with others. Educate yourself about the social, environmental, and economic impacts of food choices and advocate for ethical and sustainable food systems in your community, workplace, and beyond. By raising awareness and promoting consumer activism, you can help build a more just, resilient, and sustainable food system for future generations.

Making Environmentally Friendly Dietary Choices

Making environmentally friendly dietary choices involves selecting foods and adopting eating habits that minimize ecological impact and promote sustainability. Here are some ways to make environmentally friendly dietary choices:

1. Choose Plant-Based Foods:
- Incorporate more plant-based foods, such as fruits, vegetables, legumes, nuts, seeds, and whole grains, into your diet. Plant-based diets typically have a lower environmental footprint compared to diets high in animal products, as plant foods require fewer natural resources, produce fewer greenhouse gas emissions, and have less impact on land and water resources.

2. Reduce Meat Consumption:
- Reduce your consumption of animal products, especially red meat and processed meats, which are associated with higher environmental impacts. Consider participating in meatless meals or adopting a flexitarian diet that emphasizes plant-based foods while occasionally

including small amounts of sustainably sourced meat, poultry, fish, or dairy products.

3. Choose Sustainable Seafood:
   - Select sustainably sourced seafood options that are harvested or farmed using responsible fishing and aquaculture practices. Look for eco-labels to identify seafood products that meet environmental sustainability criteria and support healthy oceans and fisheries.

4. Minimize Food Waste:
   - Minimize food waste by planning meals, buying only what you need, storing food properly, using leftovers creatively, and composting organic waste. Food waste contributes to greenhouse gas emissions, wastes valuable resources, and exacerbates environmental degradation. By reducing food waste, you can conserve resources, save money, and minimize your environmental footprint.

5. Choose Organic and Locally Sourced Foods:
   - Select organic and locally sourced foods whenever possible to support environmentally friendly farming practices, reduce pesticide and fertilizer use, and minimize carbon emissions associated with long-distance transportation. Organic farming methods prioritize soil health, biodiversity conservation, and natural resource stewardship, promoting ecological sustainability and resilience.

6. Eat Seasonally and Regionally:
   - Embrace seasonal and regional eating by choosing foods that are in season and locally available. Eating seasonally reduces the environmental impact of food production, supports local agriculture, and promotes biodiversity conservation. Enjoying foods that are grown or produced in your region also connects you to your local food system and fosters a sense of place and cultural identity.

7. Reduce Packaging Waste:
   - Opt for foods with minimal packaging or choose eco-friendly packaging options, such as bulk bins, reusable containers, and compostable packaging materials. Minimizing packaging waste helps reduce plastic pollution, conserve resources, and protect ecosystems.

Consider bringing your own reusable bags, containers, and utensils when shopping for groceries or dining out.

8. Support Sustainable Agriculture:
- Support sustainable agriculture and regenerative farming practices that prioritize soil health, water conservation, biodiversity conservation, and climate resilience. Look for food products certified by reputable sustainability standards to ensure that your purchases support ethical and environmentally friendly farming practices.

9. Choose Fair Trade and Ethical Products:
- Choose fair trade-certified products, such as coffee, tea, chocolate, bananas, sugar, and spices, which adhere to social, environmental, and labor standards that promote fair wages, safe working conditions, and environmental sustainability in producer communities. By supporting fair trade, you can help improve the livelihoods of small-scale farmers and workers while promoting ethical trade practices and sustainable development.

10. Educate Yourself and Others:
- Learn more about the environmental impact of food choices and share this knowledge with others. Educate yourself about sustainable food systems, ethical sourcing practices, and the importance of biodiversity conservation, climate resilience, and social justice in food production and consumption. By raising awareness and promoting environmentally friendly dietary choices, you can contribute to building a more sustainable and resilient food system for future generations.